The Stop Smoking Book for Teens.

Every year some 1.5 million teenagers start to smoke. Before long many of them wish they could stop. This book takes a straight look at the physical and psychological implications of smoking cigarettes. It gives tips on quitting that young people have found helpful. A number of organized systems that help people quit are reviewed so that the reader learns just what to expect in the way of assistance. The author, himself a former smoker, offers confident and friendly advice for tackling a difficult personal problem.

Curtis W. Casewit

Photograph

The Stop Smoking Book for Teens

JULIAN MESSNER NEW YORK

Fifth printing, 1982
JULIAN MESSNER and colophon are trademarks of
Simon & Schuster, registered in the U.S. Patent
and Trademark Office.

Manufactured in the United States of America

Design by Irving Perkins

Library of Congress Cataloging in Publication Data

Casewit, Curtis W
The stop smoking book for teens.

Bibliography: p.
Includes index.
SUMMARY: Examines the physical and psychological
implications of smoking cigarettes, gives tips on
quitting, and reviews a number of organized systems
that help people quit.
1. Smoking and youth.   2. Cigarette habit.
3. Tobacco—Physiological effect. [1. Smoking]
I. Title.
HV5745.C37   613.8'5   79-27933
ISBN 0-671-33015-2

Acknowledgments

The author would like to thank the individual experts who contributed to this book. Among them are Dr. Art Ulene of NBC-TV; Dr. Sidney Werkman, the well-known psychiatrist and writer; Dr. Tommy Kofoed, Porter's Memorial Hospital, Denver; Dr. Alan Rice, Five-Day Plan; Dr. Stewart Bedford, California psychologist; Dot Springfield, American Clinics; and Pastor E. E. Christian, Denver.

Excellent help was also received from the physicians and officials of the American Cancer Society, the American Heart Association, the Office on Smoking and Health (HEW), SmokEnders, the Five-Day Plan, and other organizations.

Ben Daviss helped with additional research,

Helen Evans checked the medical accuracy, and Esther McDowell did a fine typing job.

Last, a word of gratitude to Iris Rosoff, a wise editor who understands young adults as well as writers.

CURTIS CASEWIT

Denver, Colorado

Contents

Foreword

I found myself naturally drawn to a book on how people can learn to change habits, never thinking that it might change my own life. As I mulled over statistics on the number of deaths and medical complications related to smoking, I nodded in agreement and read on to see what kind of prescriptions Curtis Casewit would offer his readers. I am happy to say that the book fulfills all my expectations and more.

The Stop Smoking Book for Teens examines everything any young adult, or older adult for that matter, needs to know about the smoking habit and how to give it up. All the accepted plans are discussed in considerable and useful detail. The problem of withdrawal symptoms, rebound eating, the use of hypnosis and behavior therapy are all covered carefully. Mr. Casewit has done an excellent job of research, and he certainly knows what he is talking about. He writes in a most direct, entertaining way. I heartily subscribe to all of his facts, concepts, and recommendations. This is an honest, straightforward book that will be valuable to young adult smokers, teachers, parents, and anyone concerned with the problem of smoking in our society.

It is simply the best compendium of ideas about smoking now available. Mr. Casewit carefully covers everything from smoking and pregnancy to the economic cost of smoking and the advantages of giving up the habit entirely. His descriptions of the bases for hypnosis and behavior therapy programs are gems of clear explanation. I have always wondered about the commercial plans advertised for smokers and now feel that I understand them quite well from the insightful descriptions given in these pages.

Teachers, parents, and community leaders can learn a great deal from this book and use it directly to develop programs that can help youngsters stop smoking. The principles described are so clearly stated that a church group or service organization could pick them up and utilize them immediately to free people from the burdens and dangers of smoking. And what a good time it is to initiate such programs. The old days, when smoking was a badge of masculinity, femininity, and sophistication, are over, and nowadays puffing on a cigarette is recognized as the dangerous, smelly act that it is.

Despite my agreement with the book's theme, I was not prepared for any personal involvement in what it had to say until I came to the part about cigar and pipe smoking. As a moderate pipe smoker (four pipes a day) and an occasional cigar smoker, I had always been comforted by the emphasis placed on the dangers of cigarette smoking as opposed to those of pipe and cigar smoking. However, when I read that pipe smokers face a higher risk of developing cancer of the oral cavity and esophagus than nonsmokers and that the danger of cancer of the larynx is three to seven times higher for these smokers than it is for nonsmokers, I realized this was not simply an interesting book I was reading. It had to do with me! The book has had its effect. I have now given up smoking altogether. I subscribe to Mr. Casewit's description of the "cold turkey" method. So I can speak not only to how well this text is written but also to how effective it is. I have always believed that books can change people's lives. Now I know that they can.

One of the peripheral benefits of this book is that it describes principles of understanding, motivation, and change that can be used to alter a host of other undesirable habits. People who have problems with eating, dependability, studying, or responsibility can use Mr. Casewit's admirably stated ideas to bolster themselves and make changes in their lives that will help them a great deal.

Reading *The Stop Smoking Book for Teens* can serve as an inspiration, a guide, and a support for anyone trying to make useful life changes. The forthcoming chapters say all that needs to be said about smoking and says it without preaching and with humor. It will interest people, and more important, it will change lives. I can give it no higher recommendation—and one I never expected to offer when I first began to study it—than to say that it works.

SIDNEY WERKMAN, M.D.
PROFESSOR OF
PSYCHIATRY
UNIVERSITY OF
COLORADO SCHOOL
OF MEDICINE
DENVER, COLORADO

Introduction

The scene is steep rock a few miles outside Estes Park, Colorado. We've been climbing since dawn. Now the sun has come up. The stone brightens. Not far from us another group moves up the stone surface, three teenagers—two boys and a girl. They are fast, yet sure climbers. Eventually, they pause on a ledge above to watch us.

I am with two well-known mountaineers. I want to experience the rock myself because I am working on a book about climbing.

The mountain face above is tricky. It tilts steeply toward the sky. There are few handholds or footholds.

I'm nervous. Out of habit, I reach into my pocket for a cigarette. I've smoked for twenty years. At that instant, faced with a difficult ascent, smoking seems the natural thing to do.

One of my companions stands a few meters above. He points the camera at me like a weapon. "Look up!" he calls.

Puffing away, I stare into his long telephoto lens.

"That won't do," he says, "for a sports book. Mountain climbers don't smoke."

The teenagers still eye us from their high perch. They have heard every word. The cigarette dangles from my lips. I suddenly realize that I not only look silly but also that I'm dangerously close to the nylon rope, my lifeline to the team. What if I burn the rope with my cigarette?

I stub it out. The young people stare at me. I have left a black mark on the eternal stone.

It is finally clear to me: *I have to quit smoking.*

Two weeks later, I actually stopped. Forever. A free clinic at a local hospital—the kind you find in every major city—helped me lick the habit. A two-pack-a-day smoker became a nonsmoker in only five evenings at the clinic.

That was ten years ago. Since then, I've written more about mountaineering. I've also done books on skiing and tennis. Without cigarettes, I feel much more at ease in these sports. I also feel better physically.

All through this period, I kept looking into the smoking problem, especially among young people. I was interested in studying tobacco smoking, not marijuana. Nor did I focus on pipe smoking or cigars. Instead, I concentrated on the cigarette habit. Because I had been addicted for twenty years myself, I understood its attractions only too well from the adult's viewpoint. But how about young smokers? How do they start? And why? What do they get out of it? Where can they obtain help to fight the addiction? What are the health dangers in a pack of cigarettes for a fifteen-year-old?

I asked doctors and other health workers many questions like these. I also looked into most organized national groups that help people quit. I went behind the scenes to see the real picture.

The current number of American smokers staggers the imagination. In one year, about 650 billion cigarettes are sold in this country. If you could lay these cigarettes end to end, you would get a path to the moon—a path as wide as a newspaper page. That paper carpet would weigh more than 2 billion pounds.

The American Cancer Society says that 53 million persons age twelve and over smoke cigarettes. About 45 million of these people would like to quit.

Unfortunately, each year, some 1.5 million teenagers *start* to smoke. Most smokers in this country start smoking before the age of twenty. Pre-teens light up too; in one California area, for instance, researchers checked up on eleven-year-olds. One in twenty smoked! It was one in five among the twelve-year-olds.

The most dramatic increase in smokers can be found among girls ages twelve to fourteen. During the past ten years, smokers in that group increased eightfold. One United States senator summed it up as "an epidemic." Obviously, smoking by young people is a serious problem. This book deals with that problem. This isn't a book that tells you what to do. It won't con you into anything, either. It's just an eye-opener.

CHAPTER ONE

Why Young People Smoke Cigarettes

"I Love Smoking"

You're in the yard of the junior high school in Santa Rosa, New Mexico. Classes are over for the day, and five kids assemble behind the building. One of the students, a blond young Anglo we'll name Billy, has been a cigarette freak since he was ten. He is thirteen now, very handsome, tall for his age. He knows many brands of cigarettes. One of his older brothers smokes, too.

Billy pulls a package of king size Winstons out of his parka pocket. He makes a ceremony of breaking the seal, neatly opening the pack, and removing a cigarette. He taps the cigarette lightly against the back of his left hand. Now Billy takes a second Winston. The other kids know the ritual. Billy tucks both smokes between his lips. He strikes a

17

match and lights first one cigarette, then the other. He gives both cigarettes to the two Spanish girls next to him. One of them has been at it for a year or so. She takes a deep drag, then sends smoke through her nostrils. Soon, the other young people are lighting up too, quietly, companionably, the gray curls of smoke unfurling into the blue southwestern sky.

This is a pleasant, mellow moment for all of them. They are away from their parents, away from their teachers. There are no hassles. The school principal has actually designated this area for smokers. He doesn't interfere with the five students plus several others who join Billy and friends.

Smoking can be a friendly act; in fact, cigarettes are offered as a gesture of hospitality in certain countries. To some of the young New Mexicans, the weed gives pleasure. "Man, I like it," Billy told me. "I don't know why. I love smoking. I get a high out of it."

Some Really Good Reasons

Smoking is a crutch for the shy person; it feels better to hold a cigarette between your fingers than just to stand there. A box of Winstons gives you something to do with your hands, and this adds to your self-confidence.

People often think they look more sophisticated or cool when they're smoking. Others admit that they first smoked as little kids to show off. Some youngsters want to do something that is forbidden.

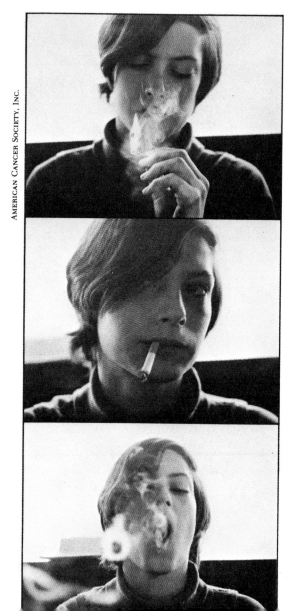

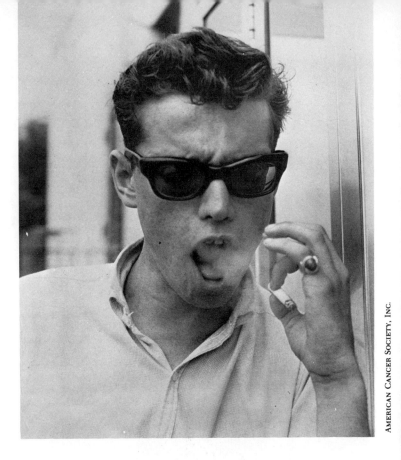

But as they grow older, they become more addicted to cigarettes. In time, they become hooked. At that point, a smoker is used to the bitter nicotine juice and to the biting, searing tobacco smoke. After some years, a smoker may even derive satisfaction from the aroma of a cigarette.

"Sublime tobacco!" wrote Byron, the English poet.

"Tobacco is divine. There is nothing to equal it!" said Corneille, the French playwright. Descriptions of the joys of smoking have appeared in the writings of famous authors. You even see well-known actors and singers photographed with cigarettes in their mouths.

Adults smoke. So why shouldn't young people?

The question makes sense. After all, doesn't everybody smoke? One important survey showed that, according to teenagers, smoking is not limited to their families and friends; it pervades the whole world around them. Teachers, executives, housewives, feminist leaders—all are thought of as smokers.

Why do people smoke? In reply to a medical column in a newspaper, the students of Franklin High School in Portland, Oregon, sent 105 letters, stating what they got out of cigarette smoking and what brought them to try it in the first place. About 24.8 percent of the school responded.

"I first tried it because both my parents are heavy smokers," wrote Becky, age fourteen. (She admitted to being hooked by now and unable to give it up.) Another Portland girl pointed to her father, who smoked "all the time" and didn't mind when she got started. She was up to seven packs a week.

Many of the Oregon high schoolers gave reasons that were similar to the attitude of the New Mexico kids in the school yard. Psychologists call it peer pressure. One of the Oregon students explained it in simpler words. "Your friends start to smoke," she wrote. "You don't want to be left out. . . ."

A recent Gallup survey showed that most teenagers start smoking at the age of thirteen. They do it to act grown up, to express independence. Some teenagers who were questioned spoke about feeling "more attractive," "taller," "more sure of yourself," or "tougher." A fifteen-year-old girl from Garden City, Long Island, New York, told an interviewer:

> At a party I can smoke a pack and a half, all in one night. Like when I'm around my friends, I'm dying for a cigarette. . . . And when I'm sad or depressed or meeting new people, I smoke a lot. A cigarette is like having company even when it's not lit.

For this girl, cigarettes were the symbol of a move from childhood to adulthood, from insecurity to security.

Just like adults, teenagers experience many pressures in their lives. Things may go badly at home or at school. Then one reaches for a cigarette. To some extent, smoking relieves anxiety.

Some young people cope with anxiety and tension in better ways. They let off steam by running or playing basketball, tennis, or other sports. They prefer soccer, table tennis, or a short tour on cross-country skis (or water skis in hot states) as a frustration fighter.

It is easy to go for a cigarette when you feel

angry or rejected. In the same sense, a smoke can console you a little when you are lonely.

A smoke can also help some people to speed things up, to stimulate their flow of adrenaline, to steady them in a crisis (soldiers traditionally get cigarettes before a battle), or to cope with a disappointment. "Some guys smoke if they feel blue," says one New York high schooler, "and maybe get rid of a downer that way."

Why Do You Smoke?

According to an American Medical Association study, there are several kinds of smokers. Which one are you? Rate yourself. (Psychologists suggest that for a week you write down your reasons for smoking.)

1. "Positive Effect Smokers"
   These are people who smoke because they obtain a pleasurable effect from cigarettes. They are of two types: those who consider smoking a stimulant and who smoke for excitement, and those who find smoking relaxing.
2. "Negative Effect Smokers"
   Such people smoke primarily to fight their feelings of distress, fear, shame, or disgust. They seek sedation rather than either stimulation or relaxation.
3. "Addictive Smokers"
   Such individuals may smoke both for

positive effect and for the reduction of negative effect to such an extent that they become psychologically addicted. They are unhappy without a cigarette and think that only a smoke will reduce their suffering.

4. "Habitual Smokers"
    Regardless of why these people started smoking, they have become so habituated that they are hardly aware when they have a cigarette in their mouths.

    A psychologist adds some more types of smokers. Rate yourself.

5. "Because-of-Others Smokers"
    These individuals justify what they do by saying, "Everyone in class smokes."

6. "Self-definition Smokers"
    These smokers fill ashtrays because they feel that smoking causes them to be "with it" or sophisticated. Such people may also explain: "A cigarette goes well with studying."

    Of course, a person may puff away for several of these reasons or may move from one to another as the habit takes hold.

The tremendous increase of smoking among teenage girls is of great concern. Since 1968, the percentage of young female smokers has actually doubled. Experts claim that the women's movement has something to do with it. Many girls equate cigarettes with freedom.

According to a U.S. government survey, the whole business also smacks of rebellion. It appears that many of the smoking girls have a streak of rebelliousness in them. One-third of the teenage smokers report that they drink to get drunk, compared to 4 percent of the nonsmokers. About 31 percent say that they have had sexual relations, while only 8 percent of the nonsmokers have done so. One-third of teenage girl smokers admit that

Some teens smoke because others do.

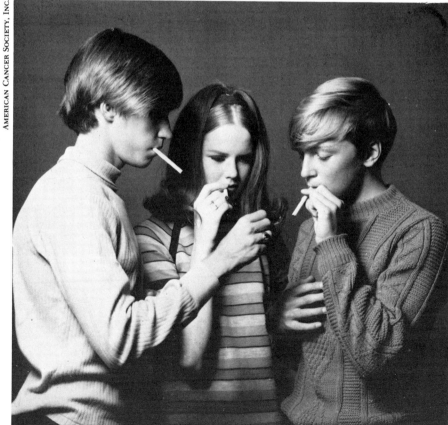

they hate school, compared to 16 percent of the nonsmokers.

A reliable national survey showed that the majority of girls were affected by the world around them. It was found that:

- Most teenage girls think of teenagers as smokers rather than nonsmokers.
- Two out of three believe that more women are smoking now than a few years ago.
- Most smoke with their parents' knowledge, and many with their parents' approval.
- Most have fathers or mothers who smoke or who once smoked.
- Most of the teenage girls who smoke indicate that their own doctors have not warned them against smoking.
- Tobacco use by females was once frowned upon, but the old taboos no longer apply. Just as the sexual code has changed, so have the restrictions against women lighting up.

The Impact of Advertising

One brand of cigarettes has welcomed these changes in the status of women by using the slogan, "You've come a long way, baby!" in its advertising. For years these particular ads showed women in tennis garb against a competition background.

(Actually almost no competitive tournament player ever smokes.)

The clever advertising people know how to please some modern women. There may be, for example, a photo of a sleek model holding up her cigarette. "Slimmer than the fat cigarettes men smoke," the ad explains. "Slim" often means "attractive."

Magazine advertising and billboards are powerful tools to sell products to teenagers. You can't ignore the sexy models in those house-high billboards. Full-page magazine ads are always in full color and make a big impression.

In addition, cigarette samples are sometimes given away. This places the product in the hands of teenagers, maybe not always directly, but certainly through an older sister or brother or a friend. Major cigarette companies also sponsor special events to promote their brands to large audiences: the Marlboro Cup Horse Race, the Virginia Slims Tennis Tournament, the Winston Cup Auto Race, the Raleigh-sponsored National Bowling Council Championship, the Kool Jazz Festival, and More's Ebony Fashion Fair. All of these make an impact on the public.

A tobacco company may shell out as much as $50 million to launch a new cigarette. In fact, the industry spent some $220 million a year on television and radio before such advertising was banned. Now it is estimated that the cost of advertising in newspapers, magazines, billboards, and other print media runs over $400 million a year.

The cigarette makers hire trained psychologists to sway you in favor of smoking their products. Some creative specialists may earn as much as $100,000 a year for convincing you that such-and-such brand is grand. Ad agencies hire the best photographers and find the most talented art directors to bring you into the cigarette camp. Ad geniuses choose enticing names for their products: "Merit," "True," "Lark," and "Real." If you are a smoker already, the ad wizards will try to engineer your switch to another brand.

Tobacco companies have fancy displays that never show dangers.   R.J. REYNOLDS, TOBACCO CO.

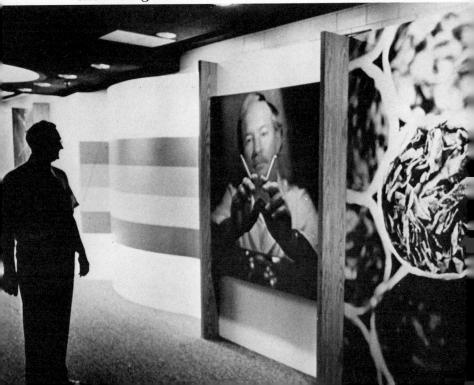

A report by the Federal Trade Commission in Washington reveals that "the trick for cigarette advertising is to associate smoking with those myriad desirable and good things which lie just beyond our reach. In a typical ad these good folks hop on and off a San Francisco cable car, smoking, singing, and smiling, finally heading downhill toward the Golden Gate and the setting sun."

According to the Federal Trade Commission, cigarette ads have three main themes:

1. Smoking and tobacco taste are satisfying.
2. Smoking is associated with desirable qualities.
3. Smoking is an activity that is free from hazard.

One brand of cigarettes makes it a point to sell not only a harmless side of smoking but also a funny one. The ads show people who bump against objects with a cigarette in their mouths. You see an artist hitting his canvas with his cigarette, for instance, or a rich lady bending her smoke against the window of her sports car. And so on.

Cigarette advertising uses only the nicest terms for a questionable product. The adjectives really get you. A cigarette is "mild" or "light," and even "mellow." Or listen to how other brands taste:

"Air conditioned!"

"A little gentler!"

"Cool!"

"Easy!"

"Delicious!"

"Friendly!"

"Smoother!"

"Soft, fresh!"

Jacquelyn Rogers, founder of SmokEnders, makes an intelligent comment about these goings-on. "The cigarette companies have done a superb marketing job," says Ms. Rogers. "Can you imagine persuading seventy million people to do something that costs a lot of money, that is kind of dirty, that makes them smell bad, that offends friends and relatives, that causes gagging and coughing and is a messy nuisance and might kill them?"

Yet the ads always link cigarettes with virile (and not weak) men, with beautiful (and never old) women. Cigarettes are also associated with healthy outdoor living. The tired cowboys in the Marlboro scenes seem to get a lift from their puffs and Salem manipulates you into thinking that a smoke is as "refreshing" as the mountain air or the scent of a forest. The Salem ad copy can really make an impression on a young mind. Two attractive people relax in a deep green landscape. "You'd enjoy smoking, too, if you smoked Salem," reads the caption under the lovely picture. The ads for Now cigarettes display a young model sitting by the ocean. "Now. It's a satisfying decision," says the caption. Some ads promise you a rich taste with lower tar; others give you some subtle signals that you'll be a success with the opposite sex if you smoke.

"The Adults Get Sick First"

In spite of all the slick advertising, you should be aware of an inscription in the left hand corner of every American cigarette ad. "Warning: The Surgeon General Has Determined That Cigarette Smoking Is Dangerous to Your Health."

How do young people feel about that statement?

A national survey assures us that most teenagers know the dangers. They have read about the horrors of lung cancer and about painful death from emphysema. Or Buerger's disease (from which you may lose a leg). Or ulcers, heart attacks, strokes. Smoking is personal pollution.

Most teenagers realize some of the dangers. Sure, you'll quit before you grow old. Besides, there is plenty of time until *you* get sick. The adults get sick first.

This attitude is understandable. A young person usually bursts with energy and feels almost immortal. It is also true that you can commit some sins against your body which would kill older folks.

Needless to say, these pages need not stop you from doing anything. You have a choice. If you want to try smoking as an experiment, then do it.

You may get hooked. One pack a week eventually becomes one pack a day. Then two or even three. As you read this, about one-fourth of the nation's teenagers are already smokers. Some of them are steering toward a period in their lives when their bodies will suffer the consequences.

You may also choose the opposite route and never start at all. If you haven't started smoking by the age of nineteen—as some psychologists state—there is a 70 percent chance that you never will.

On the other hand, you may feel that smoking is cool. If so, the next chapter will be of special interest to you.

CHAPTER TWO

What Smoking Does to You

Why That First Cigarette Doesn't Taste So Good

Ask a smoker to give you an honest answer to this question: What was it like, that first cigarette? Some people still remember it. Billy, who gets high on cigarettes now, says it openly, "The tobacco tasted bitter, but the smoke was the real bummer. First, it made me cough. Then I got dizzy. A few minutes later, I really felt sick to my stomach. . . ."

You can hear many such descriptions. Perhaps you remember some of your own early smokes, especially the high tar, nonfiltered cigarettes. The nicotine can cause vomiting and diarrhea because it is a poison. That's why some kids only smoke one or two times. They don't like it, and they never do it again.

Smoking and Sports

Any junior football or basketball player can tell you that just five cigarettes a day for only two weeks can rob you of much of your usual stamina. The best athletes—male or female—never started smoking or quickly gave it up. They can't afford to get winded.

Evidence has piled up that even your first few puffs cut into your physical performance. Smoking for some months (or years) cripples you. When I used to puff away and then try to ski the long runs of Aspen, Colorado, my irritated lungs complained. The cigarettes made me cough so violently that fellow skiers asked if I had tuberculosis. Yet I kept smoking on the ski lift. The result was that after three or four downslope ski turns, I had to stop for a rest. I was gasping for air. This had nothing to do with the Colorado altitude. My lungs just couldn't cope with the smoke.

If you happen to attend a certain stop smoking clinic, you will be shown a movie. It is about a teenage runner. You first see him circle the track three times at a fairly fast clip. The following week, after some steady cigarette consumption, the sixteen-year-old runs around the track just one time. After that—and this is a true account of a real individual—the young runner starts coughing and spitting. The tobacco has cut his energy level to the

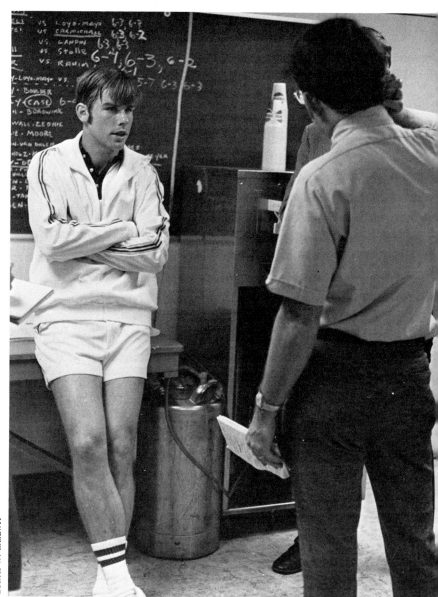

Roscoe Tanner is well known for his cool and his healthful living. He'd never smoke.

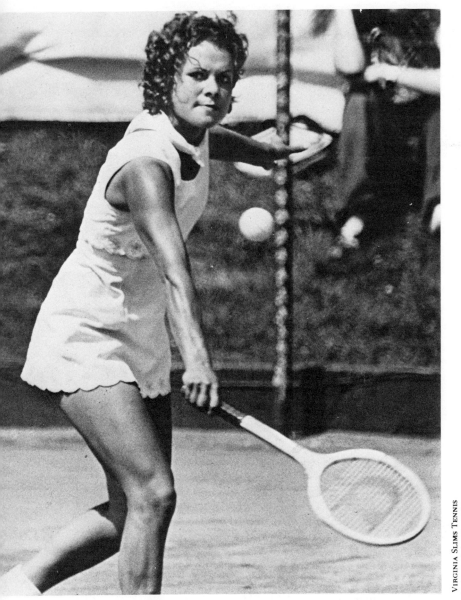

Evonne Goolagong, one of the Virginia Slims players.
Naturally, she doesn't smoke.

bone. The runner is pooped after a mere mile; he isn't getting enough oxygen.

This is not an unusual story. You can hear a similar one from squash players who can't last thirty minutes, from swimmers who cop out after half a mile. Not long ago, a young New Jersey tennis competitor told me that after she started to smoke, she had trouble winning matches against intermediates. She couldn't reach the balls in the court corners because of reduced running ability, and she never lasted longer than a set or two. A friend suggested that she stop smoking, and she did. Two weeks later, she was able to play—and win—six sets of tennis in ninety-degree heat against a strong opponent.

Dr. Kenneth Cooper, the prominent fitness expert, tested one thousand youths under the age of twenty for their physical condition. Dr. Cooper divided the young people into several groups: those who had never smoked, those who had quit, and those who were still smoking.

As you might expect, the individuals who never smoked did best in the tests, followed by those who had stopped smoking. The smokers did worst. Dr. Cooper also found that the more the athletes smoked, the worse they performed.

It takes time to become accustomed to smoking. Your body must adjust to the tremendous demand that cigarettes make on your heart, blood pressure, and circulation.

The first puffs bring a number of nasty chemicals into your mouth, throat, windpipe, and, as you smoke more and more, your lungs. Among these chemicals are propane, butane, phenol, formaldehyde, and arsenic. You also get a whiff of the pesticides used by tobacco growers.

According to the American Medical Association, more than 90 percent of cigarette smoke is composed of a dozen gases that are health hazards. The remainder consists of tars and nicotine.

Carbon monoxide, one of the smoke's most poisonous components is a colorless, odorless gas. By smoking you also breathe other lethal gases such as nitric oxide, hydrogen sulfite, nitrogen dioxide, acetone, ammonia, and acrolein. One of the worst offenders—hydrogen cyanide—assails the lining of your lungs with poisons.

Gases are easy to inhale; the particles are small enough to reach the farthest corners of your lungs. (There are about 1 billion such particles in a cubic centimeter of cigarette smoke.)

Inside Your Lungs

Turn the clock back to 1775 in London, England. Dr. Percival Pott, a noted English surgeon, gave a talk to his illustrious colleagues about a discovery he had made. Dr. Pott had discovered that chimney sweeps in their twenties to forties often suffered from lung diseases. The reason became clear: chimney sweeps started working at five years of age. Being exposed to heavy smoke all day throughout their teens affected their breathing organs. One boy of eight was found to have lung cancer.

Tobacco smoke quickly fouls up the ways in which your lungs rid themselves of foreign matter. The smoke also hits the macrophages, those "vacuum-cleaner" cells that normally remove germs and poisons. Without these protective systems in your lungs, the cigarette cloud can choke your airways and scar the air sacs, leaving behind some cancer-causing chemicals. Each year a pack-a-day smoker pours a cup of tar directly into the lungs, destroying the lungs' ability to clean themselves. The tars and acids go to work on the cells that resent incoming smoke.

The carbon monoxide that you breathe has a strong attraction for hemoglobin (which carries oxygen to your tissues). Inhaled carbon monoxide replaces vital oxygen in your blood. (Cigarette smokers have up to ten times as much carbon monoxide in their blood as nonsmokers and correspondingly less oxygen.)

There are lots of ways cigarettes affect your lungs. First of all, the smoke interferes with the normal cleansing routine of the lungs. Normally, the dust in the air around you floats onto the lining of your bronchial tubes. You might compare that lining to an escalator; it keeps carrying the dust upward via small brushes (cilia) that keep going at the rate of a thousand motions a minute. Cigarette smoke plays havoc with these hairlike structures. After a while, they can no longer function, and they leave all those foreign particles trapped in your lungs.

As you inhale more and more smoke, you also deposit a larger amount of solid tars in your lungs. In time, these tars accumulate. They also act as irritants. If they keep trickling in for a long enough period, the lung tissues begin to produce abnormal cells. Result? Cancer can begin right here.

Manchester High School West in Manchester, New Hampshire, was enterprising enough to perform some tests to prove this. The school's science teacher picked up a pair of fresh cow's lungs at the slaughterhouse. He attached the animal's lungs to a smoking machine. The science teacher then let the machine run steadily for some seventy-two hours. (This was equivalent to a few years of smoking.) The cow's lungs turned black. They developed holes, and abnormal conditions were found in the tissues. Similar things happen in humans who smoke.

Dr. Tommy Kofoed, who was a lung therapist in Greenland during the sixties and now runs Five-Day Clinics in Colorado, tells an interesting story about smoking's effect. "We never saw a case of lung cancer in Greenland. Not even one!" says Dr.

Kofoed. "The reason was obvious. Greenlanders had always been isolated. They didn't know about cigarettes. But in 1945, the first cartons arrived. After a twenty-year grace period, we had our first lung cancer case. The following year, we had five cases. Now there are many more. Reason: Greenland imports masses of cigarettes."

The statistics are even more glaring in the United States, where smoking contributes to many of the 200,000 cancer deaths each year.

Chain smokers can also wind up with chronic bronchitis. It means that they cough and spit a great deal. Cases of this ailment turn up among thirteen- or fourteen-year-olds. Smoking is also the primary cause of emphysema, a disease that destroys the lungs' air sacs. Emphysema strikes mainly smokers. One of the symptoms is difficulty with breathing. The person can barely blow out a candle and is always starved for air. "Lung cancer is a merciful death," one physican told a medical researcher. "With emphysema, you start gasping. And you may gasp for fifteen years. Until you die."

Some Other Effects

As dangerous as these chemicals are, it is the nicotine in your cigarette that really makes things happen. Nicotine, actually an alkaloid poison, acts on your adrenal glands and on your heart, releasing various stimulants into your system. Nicotine is so strong that one drop of it can kill a bird.

In seconds the inhaled smoke and nicotine:

- Start your heart pounding an extra fifteen to twenty-five beats per minute.
- Raise your blood pressure by ten to twenty points.
- Lower your skin temperature as much as six degrees Fahrenheit by cutting off circulation.
- Cause a sharp drop in your blood sugar.
- Create physical stress.
- Make your pulse race.

Soon after revving up your nervous system, the same cigarette will let you down. Suddenly, you feel fatigued. You begin to drag, and this makes you reach for another cigarette and start all over. Like a speed freak, you're up and down from now on.

Cigarettes assert themselves; you *need* them, and so you begin smoking in earnest. As you do, other mean things happen to your insides. The burning tobacco reaches temperatures up to 1,500 degrees Fahrenheit. The smoke from this burning tobacco slowly scalds and broils your insides. Burning cigarette paper poisons you with a toxic chemical known as selenite. And if this were not enough, a well-known chemist recently discovered one more fact. It seems that the atmosphere's natural radioactive particles collect on the sticky hairs of tobacco leaves. When you burn tobacco at 1,500 degrees, you send radioactive lead directly into your lungs.

The nicotine-produced adrenaline shoots fatty acids into your blood. This isn't an urgent problem for a young, healthy person. But older people pay for these fats with earlier hardening of the arteries. Cigarettes also activate your gastric juices. The burning tobacco plays havoc with your stomach lining. That's why heavy smokers eventually risk ulcers.

Cigarettes attack your gums, make your teeth yellow, and deaden your taste buds. Heavy smoking over long periods can also assault your vocal cords. In fact, cancer of the larynx (voice box) occurs almost exclusively among cigarette smokers.

Becoming Habituated to Tobacco

Teenagers who start smoking always say they can quit in a few years before it does them real harm. It doesn't work that way. The younger you are when you start, the more likely it is that you will become a regular, heavy smoker. The more you smoke, the harder it is to quit. Cigarettes become addictive.

Experts do not completely agree among themselves about whether the addiction is physical (as with morphine, for instance) or if it is only psychological and emotional. One group claims that the smoker develops a need for nicotine. It seems that nicotine causes the liver to convert stored glycogen (animal starch) into glucose (sugar). When you release sugar into the bloodstream, you get a temporary lift. Soon, the level goes down again, causing fatigue and the addicted person's craving for the next cigarette.

Nicotine addiction also affects some of the nerve cells of your brain. These physicians claim that nicotine is actually more addictive then heroin. Interestingly, once a smoker gets caught in the habit web, a certain daily amount of nicotine will become necessary to satisfy the craving for it. If he or she switches to filter cigarettes, which are weaker, the number of smokes must be increased.

Another interesting example for the physical addiction theory was found in the dog world. Scientists hooked up several dogs to a smoking machine. They were taught to smoke. After a few weeks, the dogs had become so habituated that they starting howling for tobacco.

Many experts still dispute the physiological theory, however. They say that your body doesn't crave cigarettes; the craving is in your mind. The smoking urge is purely psychological, they claim.

Here is how one doctor explains it: "Through the years the smoker forges an identical chain of habitual motions. He reaches for the pack, lifts a cigarette, lights up and inhales, smokes it to the end, and then stamps it out. The average smoker does this 30 times a day, 210 times a week, 900 times a month, 10,950 times a year."

A few cigarettes may not hurt a healthy young person. It is the cumulative effect that becomes dangerous; the cigarettes add up. When you submit your body to toxic smoke attacks day in and day out, you start to play Russian roulette with your future well-being.

The Department of Health, Education and Welfare (HEW), which has made serious studies on teenage smoking, recently released a report that was full of dark predictions. It dealt particularly with the future of females who smoke heavily. Their number keeps increasing; in the same sense, lung cancer in women has increased 400 times since 1930.

Cigarettes and Females

The U.S. Surgeon General is worried that many problems will affect young female smokers when they reach the age of forty or fifty. Unless they break the habit, which is not easy, they run an enormous risk of serious illness in those years and later. Diseases can include cancer of the tongue, windpipe, throat, bladder, or pancreas.

A recent HEW poster for high schools puts it all

on the line. It shows two girls talking to each other on a beach. One says, "Twenty-five years ago, they would have given us some dumb reasons for not smoking!"

The second girl, cigarette in hand, takes up the cue. "Sure. The worst they could say was 'Nice girls don't smoke.' Or 'It'll stunt your growth!'"

The message appears at the bottom of the color poster. It reads: "Women who smoke are dying of lung cancer and other smoking-related diseases at twice the rate of women who don't. These days there's no such thing as a dumb reason for not smoking."

It has long been known that a pack or more a day can do all kinds of unpleasant things to teenage girls. A Redding, California, skin specialist discovered that girls who smoke develop facial wrinkles much earlier in life. The nicotine makes blood vessels contract, and facial cells and tissues do not get enough oxygen. All of this helps create more wrinkles sooner.

Many medical reports have come up with even more serious evidence linking cigarette smoking and ill health. Females who take the pill and smoke more than twenty to thirty cigarettes a day eventually risk heart attacks or strokes. Doctors say that for nonsmokers of any age, the birth control pill by itself does not necessarily increase the risk of death. But for young women who smoke heavily, the pill appears to be more risky than any other

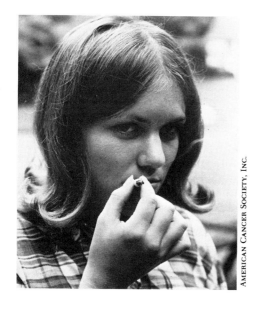

Girls face special dangers.

contraceptive method. It seems that tobacco use plus the drug increases the chances of blood clotting.

Does all this scare you? It should. These are the medical facts. Moreover, the earlier you start smoking in life, the greater the possibility of illness.

For Teenage Mothers Only

Most health hazards are shared by both males and females. But there is one which is exclusively women's—the effect of smoking on pregnancy. First of all, as you smoke, so does the other life within you. Cigarette use during the latter part of pregnancy is even more serious; the cigarettes cut down your baby's needed blood supply. As a result, the infant may weigh less than a normal one and will face a harder struggle for survival. (Some of these tiny babies die during their first week.) Gynecologists also say that heavy smoking increases the likelihood of an unsuccessful pregnancy, meaning miscarriage or infant death.

These are medically proven facts, but you won't hear them from the makers of Virginia Slims. The manufacturers are in business to sell, to make money for their stockholders. Fortunately, the companies were forced by the U.S. government to do one thing. You find it on every package and in every ad. It's the notice we mentioned: "Smoking Is Dangerous to Your Health." Not long ago, a senator went one step further. He suggested that the warning should contain more details: "Warning: Cigarette Smoking Is Dangerous to Your Health and May Cause Death from Cancer, Coronary Heart Disease, Chronic Bronchitis, Pulmonary Emphysema, and Other Diseases."

The health costs of these and other diseases are now estimated at $5.3 billion a year.

More Happenings Inside Your Body

Some people are tougher than others; they may smoke to a ripe old age and then die in a car accident. Other people happen to be almost immune to heart damage or cancer. Despite cigarettes, some people will never suffer from any lung disorders; instead, their arteries will harden fast. This often happens to smokers. Instead of dilating (enlarging) your blood vessels (as liquor does), cigarettes constrict or tighten them. The constant squeezing of your arteries, veins, and other vessels may bring about what is known as Buerger's disease. The illness is a rather uncommon but tragic one; its victims first notice leg cramping and feel pain as they walk. An inflammation can impair their blood circulation so much that they develop gangrene in a foot or leg. In some cases, the limb starts to rot and must be amputated.

I stopped smoking the first time I attended the Five-Day Clinic (about which you'll hear more later). That first night ten years ago, the physician in charge showed us a dramatic movie of a lung cancer operation. The film was shown in color. Even now, a decade later, I still see the surgeon's scalpel slicing into the patient's breathing organ. Blood spurted. Instruments make little tinkling noises. The patient in the operating room survived. Many of the people in the smoking clinic shut their eyes because they couldn't bear the sight of the surgery.

Yet staying alive is better than the 89,000 or so deaths in this country from lung cancer each year. The air pollution of cities has much less to do with lung cancer cases than smoking. One scientist suggests the following test. Unfold a clean handkerchief. Step into the street of a heavily polluted area. Take a deep breath and blow it out through the handkerchief. Now do the same experiment with cigarette smoke. According to the scientist, the cloth will be stained with tars.

Doctors state that 90 percent of lung cancer cases are caused by the personal pollution of cigarette smoking. A recent report showed that people who start smoking at fifteen are five times more likely to die of lung cancer than those who start at twenty-five.

Sure, you're young and don't think of death yet. But as you get older, you will have to face the possibility of disease.

Some high school science departments have explored the effects of the chemicals in cigarettes on animals. Perhaps you can suggest to a science teacher to build a smoking machine. This can easily be done with some lab bottles, glass tubes, aspirators, and other easily available items. Some green plants, small fish, tadpoles, frogs, and flies may be used for the tests.

Among the simplest experiments:

- Wipe the stems of several growing plants with a cotton pellet that has been saturated with tars from the smoking machine. Keep some plants as controls to observe the differences.

- Swab a cotton pellet saturated with tobacco tars on the tongue of a live frog. Note the frog's temporary collapse.
- Place a small fish in the water flask of a smoking machine. Observe how the nicotine poisoning causes the fish to roll to one side. As soon as this happens, place the fish in freshly aerated water to revive, or substitute tadpoles for fish and observe the results.
- Make a nicotine insecticide by soaking cotton pellets from a smoking machine or some cigarette tobacco in water. Test and use as spray on insects.

The experiments will convince anyone of what a few ounces of burning tobacco do to living things.

The Smoker's Heart

In time, your heart can suffer some damage from smoking, too. To be sure, a number of other factors contribute to coronary heart disease. The most important of these risk factors are high blood pressure, high levels of cholesterol in the blood, and *cigarette smoking.* Smoking can act by itself, or jointly with the other two factors, to increase the chance of developing coronary problems. One pack a day can agitate a smoker's heart to 10,000 more beats than the nonsmoker's. If you consider all that extra heart stimulation for twenty years, you can easily see what might happen. According to medical authorities, smokers suffer three times more heart attacks.

Bear in mind that smoking increases your blood pressure, which isn't beneficial either. By constricting the blood vessels, cigarette smoking makes the heart work harder. At the same time, the heart is hard up for oxygen. Evidence also points to the fact that carbon monoxide damages your most important muscle.

All this may explain why smokers risk sudden death three times more than nonsmokers. It is the smokers who account for some of the 120,000 a year cigarette-related heart attacks in the United States.

Experts tell us that the physical damage is dose-related. This means that the more you smoke (and the more you smoke high tar and nicotine cigarettes), the greater the chance of illness. There are twenty cigarettes in a pack, but if you multiply a pack-a-day habit by fifteen years, you propel a smoker into the danger zone. In other words, the damage piles up.

All these perils do disappear if a young person stops smoking. Before long, your heart beats normally again. After a few months, your lungs will look pink again and will perform. The bronchial lining will grow fresh cells, too.

That's why some of the chapters in this book will prove helpful. They will tell you how to quit. If you

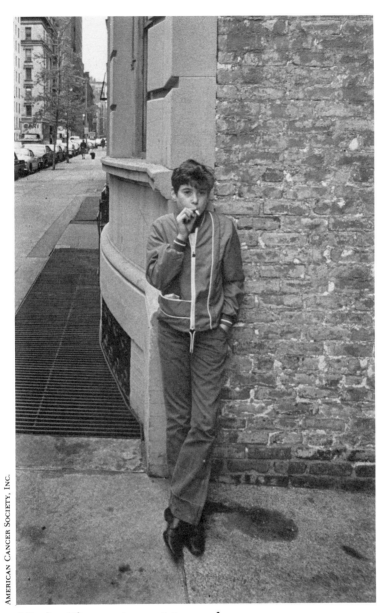

Maybe it's smarter not to smoke.

find it absolutely impossible to do, you can improve the odds slightly in these ways:

- Smoking a cigarette only halfway down.
- Never inhaling.
- Taking fewer drags.
- Buying only filter cigarettes. (Examine the packages for details on nicotine and tars, and avoid brands that contain great amounts of these poisons. You must keep your daily filter cigarette ration to a minimum.)

All these measures become difficult for a long-time smoker. Such a hooked person has a hard time making do with half of a cigarette or with one with less nicotine and fewer tars. After switching to filters, the young chain smoker (like his elders) may soon increase the number of "safe" cigarettes each day.

One New York chest surgeon sums up the problem. "The only safe cigarette is the one you don't light up," he says.

Consider another physician's words too: "You don't have to be smart to smoke, and it's smarter not to smoke."

CHAPTER THREE

How to Psych Yourself to Quit

Some Valid Reasons

Most young smokers actually want to quit. According to a HEW study, 70 percent of the young women who smoke are classified as potential quitters; they're fully aware of the health dangers. Teen-agers also know about other unpleasant aspects of smoking:

- The chain smoker's mouth never feels fresh.
- Fingers eventually show stains.
- Clothes smell of stale smoke.
- Tobacco ashes fall all over everything.

Most young smokers know the physical and material benefits of quitting:

- Better wind for swimming, cycling, tennis, ball games.

- Better all-around health. Fewer colds or coughs. No breathlessness.
- Food suddenly tastes great.
- Flowers and perfumes smell better.
- No more nicotine hangovers.
- No more holes burned in clothes or furniture.

Stopping Builds Character

Consider the true story of a wealthy writer who lived in a magnificent villa overlooking the French Riviera. A heavy smoker, he would send his chauffeur to buy cigarettes in Nice, the nearest town, which was about six miles below the man's estate. One night, the author awoke and found himself in desperate need of a cigarette. He rose and quickly realized that he had smoked an entire pack the previous evening. He looked everywhere and couldn't find any more cigarettes. The clock read three in the morning. Should he awaken his chauffeur or the other servants? The millionaire decided against it. Instead, he got dressed. He would walk to Nice himself.

But as he reached the door, he suddenly knew that it was madness to go such a long way in the middle of the night for a pack of cigarettes. He realized with a pang that he had become enslaved to a habit. He, a successful and wealthy man, was totally dependent on tobacco. That quiet night, he asked himself some important questions. Was he really a strong man? Or did dependence on cigarettes make him a weakling? Real strength of character meant he would have to give up cigarettes.

The man analyzed the pros and cons until dawn broke. As the sun came up, the wealthy author knew that he faced a challenge. He had smoked all through his adult life. It would be difficult to quit.

But he would. And he did right then and there.

True independence means that you can say, I choose *not* to smoke. I do have a free choice. I am not a slave. I want to control my own life.

Smoking Isn't "In" Anymore

Cigarettes may be the fashion with your peer group. A pack of Virginia Slims may look chic in an ad. By the same token, you rarely see a top *Vogue* or *Harper's Bazaar* model photographed with a cigarette. This used to be fashionable until the early fifties. Now most sophisticated women are into physical fitness instead. Many other people— explorers, mountain climbers, surgeons, athletes, environment experts—have long given up tobacco. Today you do not see as much smoking as you used to among large gatherings of physicians who specialize in internal medicine; these specialists know the risks.

Dr. John F. Knight, an advisor to the U.S. gov-

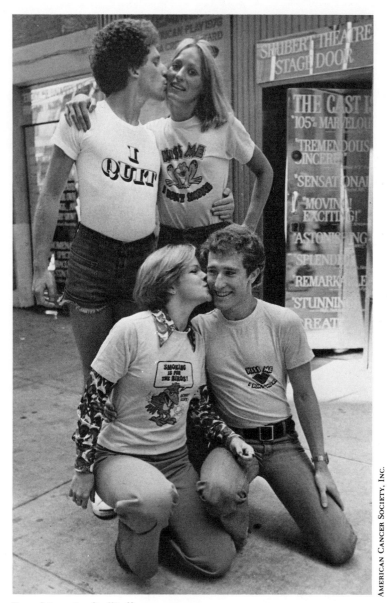

Smoking isn't "in" anymore.

ernment, puts it this way: "Smoking isn't 'with it' anymore! Despite what the advertisers say, telltale statistics show a different story. Many smart people, and people considered avant-garde, no longer regard smoking the way they once did. In fact, it's definitely old hat for those who want to stay alive, feel bright, and remain mentally alert for the major part of their waking day."

A government study of teenage smokers came up with the data that few A students smoke while many C and D students do. Most college students at the best universities no longer indulge, either. Take Princeton University, for instance. Rated as one of the finest colleges in the world, Princeton was always hard to get into; the classes attracted only the brightest young people. Eight years ago 45 percent of Princeton University's undergraduate students smoked cigarettes. This year, the percentage is down to 6.9.

An interesting situation exists at one western college. Most of the University of Colorado students became so angry with their peers who smelled up the cafeteria with smoke that they formed a special committee of vigilantes. Non-smoking volunteers would keep an eye out for anyone who lit up. The smoker would be approached and asked to put out his or her cigarette. If the smoker refused?

A student tells what happened next. "J. confronted me while I was sitting at a table having my first cup and cigarette of the day—poor timing—and proceeded to attempt to intimidate me into putting out my cigarette. When I refused, he whipped out his water gun and zapped my cigarette while shouting to everyone in the cafeteria that all smokers were doomed to the same treatment!"

This may be a little extreme, but it illustrates a point. At some schools, the smokers are left in peace, but they are counted. A Harvard University poll, for instance, shows that only 2 percent of the freshmen smoke cigarettes. At Dartmouth College, smokers have become equally rare.

In fact, cigarette consumption is down for adults these days. Since 1964, when the U.S. Surgeon General confirmed the lung cancer research of the American Cancer Society, there has been a continuing decline in the percentage of adult smokers in America.

In 1964 a majority of all men in their thirties were cigarette users. Now the number of males is only 38 percent, and the same is true for men and women in most age groups. To the dismay of the tobacco industry, fewer young Americans between the ages of twenty-one and twenty-five smoke cigarettes than fifteen years ago.

All this also explains why you sometimes find yourself in an office or public place where you spot a sign that says, "Thank you for not smoking." Or why some young people drive cars with bumper stickers that read, "Kissing a Smoker Is like Licking an Ashtray."

Disadvantages of Being a Smoker

Not smoking is now in. You may experience this trend in your own high school. The regulations in a number of schools reflect the new approach.

Seventh and eighth graders at Tahanto High School in Boylston, Massachusetts, must get permission from their parents before they can smoke in school. In addition, the principal has restricted smokers to a designated outdoor area during three periods in the day. The periods will be discontinued if students keep smoking inside the school.

In San Bernadino, California, the board of education decided to expel students caught smoking, since suspending students for smoking violations had not worked in the past.

In Ridgewood, New Jersey, both the faculty and students of a local high school voted to ban all smoking in the building after a biology class showed people the effects of carbon monoxide.

In Chicago, at Foreman High, students caught smoking in the school building receive an automatic three-day suspension.

As you look around your community, you will find that many hospitals forbid the sale of cigarettes in their shops and other hospitals ban smoking altogether. On commercial airliners, the smokers are separated from the nonsmokers.

Smoking has become illegal in many public places; in others, like theaters and restaurants, smokers are assigned a special area.

As you embark on a career, you'll quickly note that many prospective employers are against smoking cigarettes. With such employers, smoking during an interview means that you're out before you're even in. Take a well-known Denver, Colorado, oilman who recruits eighteen- to twenty-two-year-olds for outdoor work. He says frankly that he is a health freak and would never hire a young smoker. This also makes sense, of course, because some of his crews work in areas where fires could start. Some fire departments (like a typical one in Alexandria, Virginia) won't hire smokers.

When you leave home and rent your first apartment, you will meet more and more landlords who refuse to rent to smokers. The building owners not only dislike the pollution, but they're also afraid of fires. Many fires can be traced to someone who fell asleep with a cigarette; other fires are caused by smokers who get drunk.

The national statistics say a lot in this regard. National Fire Protection Association files, for instance, show that more than half of all fatal residential fires are the result of cigarette smoking.

According to the NFPA, during a recent year more than 137,000 fires were smoking-related. That's more than one fire every four minutes! Property losses from those fires were estimated at more than $166 million.

A major fire in Santa Monica, California, was reported in many newspapers because several teenagers were involved in it. The fire started when a teenage boy fell asleep in his bed while smoking a cigarette. Soon, the frame house was completely ablaze. The boy died in that fire. Two of his younger sisters died, too. A third sister suffered burns so severe that she was in pain for a full year.

Consider the Costs

You might psych yourself to stop smoking by figuring out how much money you really waste on your habit. Some of the 30 million quitters gave financial reasons for stopping.

Even one pack a day costs a lot in the long run. At only fifty cents a day, you pay $3.50 a week, or $14 a month, $183 a year. That's the minimum. If you live in certain states or Canada, you can pay much more than that. You must also increase the amount you spend if you buy your packs from a machine. Cigarette machines at better restaurants, for instance, are real rip-offs. If you become a chain smoker—and there's a good chance you will unless you quit—you must expect other expenses. You will burn holes in your best clothes, for instance. You may want to buy a lighter which requires flints. Unless you can get free matches, you will have to put out money for them too.

Could you make good use of $200 a year? You save that much skipping that pack a day.

Some young people eventually graduate to two packs a day. So if you move on to forty cigarettes a day, you set fire to about 400 one-dollar bills a year. In ten years, that's $4,000. In thirty years, you've burned up $12,000 worth of cigarettes. City, state, and federal taxes add to the expense and keep going up. (In Sweden, for instance, where a pack costs $2.00, the government puts a heavy tax on cigarettes to discourage smokers). You can find better use for your hard-earned money: good camping gear, a backpack, clothes, a vacation, some expensive stamps for your collection—all are possibilities if you stop smoking.

Adults can save not only on the costs of the cigarettes but on other items as well. Insurance, for instance, is often cheaper for nonsmokers than for smokers. A number of companies pay a bonus to workers who quit smoking. A printer in St. Louis, Missouri, for example, who lost many employees to lung cancer, now offers $500 to anyone who quits. The check is presented after a two-month period of not smoking.

See Yourself as a Nonsmoker

Psychologists recommend a change of attitude. They say that from now on, you should see yourself as a nonsmoker. There are many ways to do this.

First of all, you can model yourself after people who are nonsmokers. These people may be in your own school, achieving the highest grades or getting acclaim in other ways. (A high school in Chester, Pennsylvania, actually posted photos of important, popular students who didn't smoke.)

You can also observe those people you admire in the world around you. This may be an extremely successful, attractive, physically fit relative or friend.

Some young people search for models among famous people in various fields:

- Actor Tony Curtis decided to quit and did.
- Actress Rosemary Harris, famous for her Broadway and television appearances, quit; she is now a proud nonsmoker.
- Dick Button, international figure skater, television producer, and commentator, gave up the habit.
- Bob Mathias, Olympic gold medal decathlon winner, pushes nonsmoking.
- Conductor-composer Leonard Bernstein, admired for introducing classical music to young people, won a long battle against cigarettes.

- Joseph Califano, a lawyer who has held several high-ranking government offices, asked his son what he wanted for his birthday. "Quit smoking, Dad," the son said. Califano did.
- Best-selling mystery novelist Robert Harrington stepped in front of a mirror one day. He didn't like the pallor of his face. He looked like a sick man. He quit.

"Begin to associate with people who devalue smoking," says one psychologist. "If people smoke, study them closely. Listen. Note the choking coughs. Spot their tar-stained fingers. Ask yourself if these are your models." Another expert goes one step further. He suggests that you observe your own father if he smokes. Listen to him wheeze. Listen for his early morning cough. Surely, you can do better.

Taking That First Step

There are basically two ways to quit.

One: You stop gradually. You begin by cutting down. This is called "tapering off."

Two: You stop suddenly. You stop completely. The sudden quitting is known as "cold turkey." It means that you are through; you will not smoke even one more cigarette.

Either way, you will have to overcome some obstacles.

Whether you smoke only five to ten cigarettes a day, like most teenage smokers, or a whole pack, you will need some willpower.

Not everyone has willpower. But *you* are the one who must decide that you really want to give up cigarettes.

Even wanting to quit will not guarantee success. You may not stop on the day you'd hoped to. Perhaps you face an emergency after you've quit, and you go back to another pack. Or someone offers you a cigarette, you take it, and you must start the fight all over.

There is nothing wrong with failure, especially if you try again. Mark Twain's famous and witty words express it best of all: "To cease smoking is the easiest thing I ever did. I ought to know because I've done it a thousand times!" It isn't easy to battle an addiction, so don't worry about not succeeding right away.

Fortunately, young people find it much easier to quit than adults. After all, adults have been smoking for a longer time, and twenty-year habits are harder to break than two-year habits. In fact, it should be a cinch to give up cigarettes if you have only tried them for a few weeks.

Adults and young people have one thing in common, however. Both need a motivation to stop.

What would be your reasons? Try to write them down before you start a fight which may demand a lot from you.

As you sit down to compile your list, you might think about the statistics given out by the Surgeon General's office, the American Cancer Society, the American Heart Association, and other organizations.

Review the facts that you know about the risks. Remind yourself that if you continue smoking, you may lose six and one-half years of your life, that your chances of dying between twenty-five and sixty-five years of age are twice as great as those of the nonsmoker. Would you fly in an airplane if the risk of crash and death were even close to the risks of cigarette smoking? Think over the reasons why you should not smoke: the risk of disease, the tastelessness of food, the cost, the cough, the bad breath, the mess and smell of the morning after.

Your list can also include some psychological motives. Many people quit smoking because they prefer to be in charge of their lives; they hate to be enslaved. They want to be master of their own fate. Psychologists say that knowing your own motivations will help you gain the strength necessary to stop. Many scientists see quitting as an exercise in self-mastery, one that introduces a new dimension of self-control. You'll feel proud afterward.

On another sheet of paper, write down the plus factors of smoking. Ask yourself these questions:

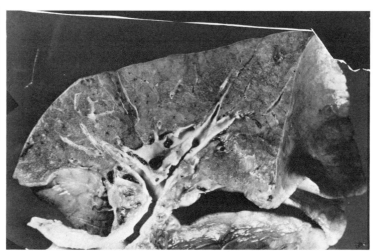

A photograph of a normal human lung.

A photograph of a cancerous human lung.

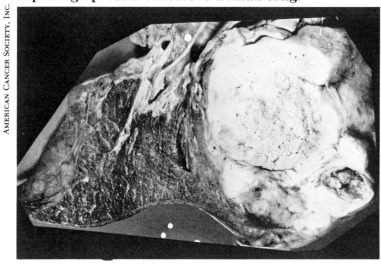

What do I really get out of smoking? What are the benefits?

By now, you will also have an insight into how strongly you feel about quitting. One clinic asks you to ask yourself:

How important is quitting to you?

1.   Is it urgent?
2.   Is it a matter of life and death?
3.   Is it very important?
4.   I should do it, but there isn't any rush?
5.   I was talked into coming here, and I'm not sure I want to go through with it?

The answer should really prove helpful to you.

Tapering Off

Many health experts say that gradual quitting for young people who smoke less than half a pack a day is okay. Tapering off can get you off cigarettes altogether. However, for a teenager who started smoking at age ten and who now must buy a pack a day, the cold turkey method would be better.

In either case, you will have to pick the right date for your program. It would be unwise, for instance, to start reducing your tobacco intake if your parents are just splitting up, or if you face major exams in school. If you will be attending a party with friends who smoke heavily and expect you to smoke also, this would not be the easiest time to stop.

In any case, remember that it's *your* choice. Only you can do it. According to Dr. J. W. McFarland, who codeveloped the famous Five-Day Plan, you should not become discouraged if things don't work out immediately.

You may fail to cut down and go back to your regular tobacco ration each day. But by having already chosen to stop, you've strengthened your willpower. Thanks to your new dormant strength, your second or third try *will* succeed.

Youth experts suggest that you begin by smoking one less cigarette a day. Make each cigarette a special decision and put off making that decision. Say to yourself, "I won't light up from five to six o'clock while doing my homework."

Other specialists say that you might start smoking one hour later each day. Tapering off should be carried out according to the rules you set for yourself. Perhaps you will skip not only the school smoking breaks, but your usual afternoon puffs as well. Instead, you decide that you've earned a cigarette at only seven o'clock.

All along, you should consult the lists you've made. Psychologists further recommend keeping track of each cigarette you consume and at what time you smoke it. One system of quitting suggests that you eliminate all but perhaps three "hard-core" cigarettes a day. Then cut these out, too.

Stopping becomes easier if you spend time in places where you can't smoke, such as libraries, buses, theaters, certain offices, swimming pools, and department stores.

You can also summon the willpower to quit cold turkey on your own. For some young people, this is easier than for others.

As you cut down from ten to five cigarettes a day, you will begin to move toward Q Day. Tapering off often leads to quitting for a day, and then completely.

People use various tricks to help them quit smoking:

- They no longer buy a carton of cigarettes; they buy only one pack at a time.
- They smoke only a third of each cigarette.
- They keep an unlighted cigarette between their lips.
- They light one, place it in the ashtray, and leave it there.
- They never carry matches.
- They remove ashtrays from their home.

The American Cancer Society suggests that you can reduce your daily intake by making your cigarettes hard to reach. If you have one pocket in which you always carry a pack, put the pack in another so that you will have to fumble for it. If you use your right hand to bring the cigarette to your mouth, try using your left hand. Is it your custom to dangle the cigarette in the right corner of your mouth? Try the left side.

It should require real effort to get to a cigarette. Wrap your package in several sheets of paper, or place it in a tightly covered box. If you leave your change at home, you won't be able to use a cigarette machine. Shift from a brand you like to an unappealing brand. None of these devices will work, however, if you're not sure *why* you should quit. Psychologists insist that you must know your own reasons and you need to repeat them to yourself every day at least once.

Psyching Yourself to Quit Completely

The tapering off method should lead you to Q Day. According to the latest figures, about 95 percent of the smokers—young or old—manage to quit by themselves. Only about 5 percent need a group to help them. On the other hand, it may be easier to stop with the help of a group. You'll read more about groups in the next chapter.

According to B. F. Skinner, a well-known psychologist, the cold turkey method is the best one. To break a habit slowly is much harder, claims Dr. Skinner. For the young smoking addict, tapering off might be almost impossible. Such a person must quit abruptly.

Young athletes won't find it particularly difficult to give up cigarettes from one day to the next. The approach of a big interscholastic tennis tournament or ski race will surely help. It also helps to have a coach who threatens to kick you off the team if he ever catches you smoking again. The basketball player, the serious swimmer, and the young runner have an advantage over other young people who don't like sports. They have to stop smoking to play well.

Q Day: You Need Timing

Good timing is of great importance if you are to stop smoking. A Denver, Colorado, teenager's timing was excellent. He was cured of cigarettes the day his parents took him on an ocean cruise along the Mexican coast. "I still smoked on the drive to the West Coast," he admits. "But I'd made up my mind that boarding our ship would be the right moment. So I threw my last half-pack into the sea. Then I walked up the ship's gangplank. This was it! Never smoked after that. And had a great time in Acapulco. . . . "

It may be weeks or even months between your I-choose-to-quit decision and the actual moment when you quit. One Michigan boy, for instance, made up his mind in August that he would smoke his last cigarette on Christmas Eve. And he did.

Many teenagers picked New Year's Day or another holiday when they were relaxed. Your birthday offers an excellent possibility; after all, that is the day on which you start a new year in your life.

According to the American Cancer Society's "I Quit Kit," probably the best situation is one in which you would not be too tempted to smoke. But maybe you'd rather wait for a tougher situation, like a meeting or a party. This gives you a chance to test yourself.

Pretend there's a "No Smoking" sign around. Don't smoke for as long as you're in that particular situation. Once you know that you can control your urge in one instance, try others. You'll find that in many situations when you feel you just must have a cigarette, you really don't need a cigarette at all.

One ACS doctor says, "If you can get through the first day, the next will be easier, and easier, and easier. Until after a while the urge to smoke will leave you, and you'll wonder why you didn't quit years ago."

The battle isn't over yet, though, and you should be very wary. Avoid the patterns that connect you to the habit—like the school yard smoking break with a peer group. Do something else while the cigarette freaks are out there. Go to the library instead, or talk to a teacher.

Clyde Jones, an Oklahoma-born tennis player and former four-pack-a-day smoker, says that the first day is the hardest. But Jones split his cold turkey morning into thirty-minute segments. "That's really helpful," Jones explains. "After the first half hour, you say to yourself, 'Okay, now another half hour.' And you'll do it." Jones suggests that after one hour, you say, "Okay, now one more hour." And so on through the day. You'll feel great.

The First Few Days

The experts who work out the stop smoking systems have researched your next steps with great care. Some of the recommendations are simple. Among the most important ones are these:

- Breathe deeply. Breathe each time you feel the craving to smoke. Take at least ten deep breaths three times daily.
- Hide all evidence of cigarettes—ashtrays, matches, and so on—so you aren't reminded of your habit.
- Lay in a supply of chewing gum, cough drops, carrot sticks, and fruit. This is the time to allow yourself some real treats.
- Drink plenty of water. Doctors recommend at least six glasses a day. Some experts suggest orange juice or other fruit juices.
- Exercise as much as you can. Take up a new sport or participate in sports you like.

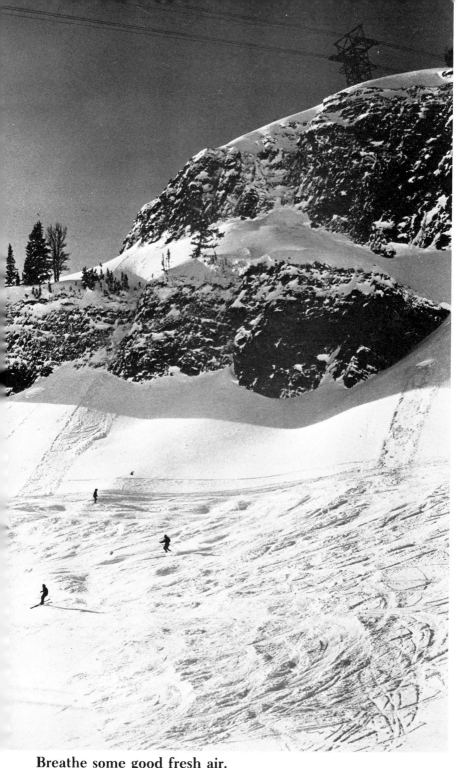

Breathe some good fresh air.

- Obtain seven or more hours of sleep daily.
- Provide time for recreation. Try to take some of this recreation out-of-doors.

For some people, those first few days will be the toughest. You may need to be prepared for the battle that goes on inside you. If you have smoked for a long time, you will miss the presence of the cigarette between your fingers and the almost automatic movements of your hands. One psychologist figured out that an habitual smoker, in a year's time, will actually move the hand to the mouth some 40,000 times during a year. Compare the smoker to a driver. Both are programmed by habit. The driver shifts gears automatically. The smoker automatically lights up, inhales, flips the ashes, and moves the cigarette toward the lips. All these actions are now part of the habit.

So what do you do? Some people reach for a pencil instead, and they compute the money they've saved so far. One health worker advises that when the impulse to smoke is strong, you should try a substitute: a drink of water, a piece of candy, a walk around the block, stretching, and deep breathing.

These substitutes may only satisfy you temporarily, but they will keep you alert and aware and will lessen the strength of your desire to smoke. Equally important are constant reminders to yourself of why you are giving up cigarettes. Remember the reasons that you listed for not smoking? Recall the basic data about disease and disability caused by cigarettes. Remember your own special reasons for quitting.

After you stop smoking, you may expose yourself to some needling by schoolmates. Consider what they are really saying. Maybe they are envious. They would like to stop, too, but they can't.

During the first few days, your I-choose-not-to-smoke decision can be strengthened in various psychological ways. An Illinois student, age eighteen, made a bet with a friend. He bet five dollars that he could get along without tobacco for two weeks. He won. In another instance, a Wyoming girl made a wager with her boyfriend. She bet she would quit. If she did, he would have to buy her dinner at Cheyenne's best restaurant. That is exactly what happened.

Some psychologists also believe that it is a good idea for you to tell others about your decision. Tell your parents, who will give you support. Tell your girl friend or boyfriend. Tell a favorite teacher, someone you particularly like or respect. This will make you want to live up to your resolve. A public commitment strengthens your willpower.

Group action helps, too.

In the next chapter, we will find out how group action works and where to get help, in school and outside.

CHAPTER FOUR

Where to Get Valuable Help

School Programs

In order to quit smoking, you don't have to rely solely on your own inner resources. You can get outside help, too, not only in major cities through some well-known programs, but in school, too.

Various government agencies, some private organizations, hospitals, and churches concentrate on helping young people. Experts in the Department of Health, Education and Welfare are truly concerned; they know that the future health of the nation is at stake. These people look twenty years down the road and see today's teenage smokers as tomorrow's lung cancer statistics. Large sums of money are therefore being poured into the battle against teenage cigarette smoking. Perhaps you've seen the posters, read one of the pamphlets, or viewed some of the films.

The campaigns take many forms, and there are many sponsors. In New England, for instance, the Lung Association may supply your science teacher with some unusual equipment that monitors your heart rate, skin temperature, and the carbon monoxide in your bloodstream. The classroom tests really open the smokers' eyes.

In Denver, Colorado, and other major cities, the excellent Five-Day Plan leaders come to junior and senior high schools as part of the health education curriculum. During a few fascinating hours, you'll be made aware of the problems caused by nicotine. A doctor will give slide shows and show films to the class. These will be followed by frank discussions. There is no charge for these worthwhile sessions. The leaders make no attempt to change you from a nicotine and tar dependent into a nonsmoker. That wouldn't be possible in a few hours. Instead, you get a good look at smoking, and you learn that it's possible to give it up. In addition, you find out where to turn for help.

In Florida and elsewhere, the local chapter of the American Cancer Society may send a representative to your school to make various presentations. One cancer society chapter in Florida produced a fifteen-minute videotape for schools with the title, "Smoke–Choke–Croak." It made a lot of people think.

In other cities, the ACS organizes groups of eight to eighteen persons to meet twice a week for four weeks. They meet in churches and hospitals, where volunteer therapists lend a hand. California alone saw 50,000 people go through these free ACS clinics during the past five years. You will see movies, get a "buddy" (male or female) to discuss your progress with, and you will learn a lot about yourself.

In some states, the staff from a local hospital may come to visit your school. The St. Helena Hospital and Health Center in Deer Park, California, developed a high school smoking cessation program at the request of the Napa Valley school system. To give students an incentive to take the course, one hour of credit was offered for fifteen hours of classroom work. Participants attended the antismoking program for one hour each day for three weeks. As part of the course, students designed elementary school antismoking program curricula and then traveled around the school district speaking to students about smoking.

Teachers and school nurses in more than two hundred school districts in twenty-eight states have received training from the National Clearinghouse for Smoking and Health. For a period of several weeks, young adults take a close look at the human respiratory system and the lungs. The teenagers become familiar with the heart and circulatory system. In the seventh grade, the students examine the brain and nervous system. You hear a great deal in these sessions about the effects of smoking. What's more, you receive a free "Teenage Self-Test" which gives you some new insights. (You can also order the kit by mail. See addresses at end of this book.)

In some cities, the Lung Association as well as the Heart Association or the PTA may get into the act. In many areas of the country the Department of Health, Education and Welfare has developed special programs for teenagers. They may consist of lectures, television shows, videotapes, or give-away kits. All these are free. State health departments or state health agencies may also be organizing some withdrawal clinics. You can ask any local hospital for information about addresses and times.

Getting Help from Large Groups

Some individuals function better when they obtain support from a group. If an entire class of thirty young people decide to quit together, the individual no longer has to battle the habit alone. Instead, he or she can do so in company.

Group action works especially well when the people have one common aim. Many such cessation sessions are headed by experts in the field, including physicians, psychiatrists, psychologists, social workers, and nurses.

Such stop smoking clinics can only work, though, if you faithfully attend all the sessions. This takes discipline. You are expected to pay attention and to follow through after the sessions as well.

The director of one typical clinic explains her expectations this way:

- Sincerity and depth of motivation are basic ingredients necessary to make the program work for you.
- Be on time or a few minutes early for every session.
- Follow our instructions to the letter. Total success depends on maintaining the precise timing sequence that has worked for thousands of others.
- Keep in touch. Answer our follow-up queries promptly. We want to know how you're doing.

Many programs are available outside your school; these will be more goal-conscious. Clinics take place in the evening, at little or no cost.

A free teenage withdrawal clinic was held in York, Pennsylvania, with the help of the Tuberculosis and Respiratory Disease Association. Literature, speakers, and films attracted forty-five students, of whom thirty-four stopped smoking. The clinic lasted five days.

You may obtain group help on weekends or during certain weekday afternoons. Smokers are at first leery about any withdrawal programs. One group leader summed up the questions that come up most frequently:

- Will it work?
- Will I climb the walls?
- Will it cost money?
- Will I be embarrassed or humiliated?
- Is the program accepted in the community?
- Will I gain weight if I stop smoking?

Although most stop smoking clinics are meant for adults, a teenager is generally welcome. In addition, there are commercial clinics that cost money. Whatever your age, keep in mind that the organizers won't turn down a paying customer. In the same sense, psychologists, hypnotists, and other experts can assist you privately with their methods. (You'll learn about the more expensive programs in the next chapters.)

The Five-Day Plan

Let's assume that some time ago you tried to taper off. Your aim was to smoke only a couple of cigarettes a day. But you slid back to ten a day. You next tried the sudden stop or cold turkey method. You even picked a good time. You had a severe cold with a runny nose that made cigarettes taste like garbage. You quit smoking only long enough to regain your usual good health.

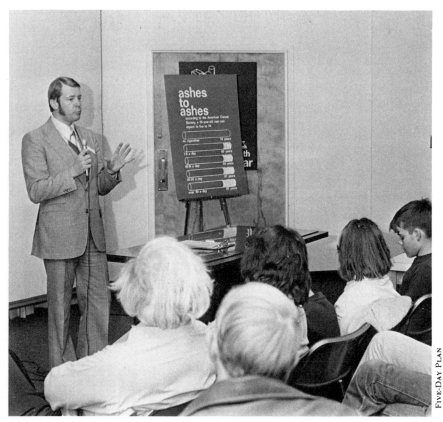

Dr. Tom Kofoed of the Five-Day Plan in Denver speaking before a group.

Now you feel fine. And you're back to ten or more Winstons a day.

You know that you need another Q Day. So what do you do?

You could ask your parents for help. Perhaps they know a cessation system which they could share with you. Unfortunately, this doesn't always work out too well. Even if you're on good terms with your folks, they may get a little impatient with you. It is like learning to drive. Sometimes an outsider—a professional driving instructor—can achieve better results than your own father or mother. The same applies to smoking.

If you really want to stop, consider a professional clinic. The clinic would involve a group of people, perhaps be organized by a hospital, and be non-profit.

The Five-Day Plan to Stop Smoking might be the best bet for a young person. The plan has become international. It is run by dedicated, motivated health workers—physicians, medical specialists, psychiatrists, health advisors—who volunteer their services. Your cost is no more than what you would pay for a few cartons of cigarettes. Up to now, about 13 million persons have used the plan. Around 85 percent of these people kicked the cigarette habit. Time involvement? Only a few evenings.

How the Plan Works

At this point, you may wonder what the plan is all about.

The scene is Porter's Memorial Hospital, in South Denver. It is Sunday evening, around seven o'clock. The smokers arrive one by one at a special desk, where a nurse welcomes them.

You register and file into the small hospital auditorium.

Men and women, boys and girls, of all ages, all faiths, ethnic backgrounds, and educational levels are represented here. Whoever you may be, the group will have an effect on you. The other people are in the same boat; so you can count on group support.

The man in charge is Dr. Tommy Kofoed. He is in his thirties, a runner, cross-country skier, and swimmer.

This former lung therapist understands smokers.

Dr. Kofoed has many colleagues around the country. As he speaks with you in Denver, other clinic directors address smokers in Orlando, Florida; Madison, Tennessee; Fort Worth, Texas; Hinsdale, Illinois; Shawnee Mission, Kansas; Deer Park, California, and many more locations.

On the first evening, Dr. Kofoed will explain the Five-Day Plan. "The sharing and learning experience begins tonight," says the Five-Day Plan leader. "You will hand over your cigarettes. I know this sounds scary. What's more, you will choose not to smoke for the next twenty-four hours. . . . "

In Denver, you will be shown a humorous film about a man who wakes up every morning with a cough. The trials and tribulations of this smoker make you laugh.

Other Five-Day Plan hospitals may show a color film of a lung cancer operation. There is no humor at all in that movie. The Five-Day Plan director won't admit it, but the film—by the American Cancer Society—is meant to frighten you. In fact, many young and old smokers are cured right then and there. (The author was one of them.) You also receive some psychological help at the clinic. You learn to say, "I choose not to smoke."

The emphasis is on *you*. No one tells you what to do. No one makes you stop. You choose to stop. You choose your reason for quitting.

The method works well. In fact, the plan has been tested for twenty years. The slogan, "I choose not to smoke," has become an important part of the clinic. It says something about a personal choice. You stop because you personally decided to, not because your parents hassled you.

Since smoking is often based on rewarding yourself, the plan teaches that you can substitute something else for the weed. Orange juice, for example. Every time you crave a smoke, you drink a glass of juice instead. Pure orange juice is healthful, and it replenishes vitamin C, an important point for smokers. In a way, the juice becomes a substitute for the cigarette, and it tastes much better.

The Five-Day Plan organizers also recommend plenty of fresh fruit during those critical twenty-four hours. Treat yourself to all kinds of things like fresh berries, pineapple, bananas, grapes. Avoid spicy meals and drink milk instead of coffee. Stay away from beer, wine, and liquor, even if your school companions offer you some. Alcohol, coffee, and peppery dishes make people want to smoke.

Group Power

Although the other people who join you for the Five-Day Plan are strangers at first, you will soon feel their influence. You exchange telephone numbers so that you can talk to others when the craving for a cigarette becomes too strong. At the end of the meeting, the entire group is encouraged to throw away all cigarettes. (A large cardboard container is ready for that purpose.) You do it together; this is called group dynamics. A young person will feel good about the group spirit because so many people are in their late teens or early twenties.

During your second evening meeting, which lasts only ninety minutes, some people announce that they have indeed quit. Well, if they can do it, surely you can, too. The buddy system also encourages you to call someone in the group. Friendships develop. When things get rough that week and you feel a great urge to smoke, you can enlist the help of other Five-Day members.

At each session, more and more smokers hold up their hands. Yes, they bought no more cigarettes. Yes, they discarded the ashtrays. Yes, they quit abruptly. They are making do with juices (no alcoholic beverages, ever!) and with taking deep breaths. There is something contagious about these Five-Day members announcing their success.

You are repeatedly impressed by the excellence of the speakers. You listen to the voices of authority. A gynecologist talks about smoking and pregnant women. A dentist reveals the dental results of smoking. A heart specialist tells you all without holding back. A psychologist helps you with your own struggle.

You see a terrifying film on emphysema. You listen to former smokers who speak about their happy lives without tobacco. Nutritionists meanwhile give you some advice on how not to get fat after you regain your sense of taste. You see an excellent film on running.

Directors in some cities vary their presentations a little. In one community, for instance, you meet well-known sports figures who tell that they have quit. Elsewhere, you may hear a speaker who makes a different impact. It could be a man who comes with an oxygen tank. He is still suffering from emphysema. Another ex-smoker lost his speech after forty-five years of addiction; doctors removed his voice box because of cancer. It isn't easy to ignore such people.

You also get a personal control booklet. In brief, it tells you:

- How to relax.
- How to avoid familiar spots or activities that might lead to a smoke.
- When to exercise and how to breathe.
- What to eat and drink during the five days.

The result of all this seems remarkable. In Denver, 90 percent of the smokers, including the young people, stopped for good. Nationally, the figure is between 80 to 90 percent. All for the price of a few cartons of cigarettes.

Behind the Five-Day Plan

The Five-Day Plan was developed in the early 1960s by J. Wayne McFarland, M.D., and a Seventh-Day Adventist clergyman, Elman J. Folkenberg. The plan was copyrighted in 1962 and has been maintained and directed ever since from the church's world headquarters in Washington, D.C. The courses are backed by local physicians, health agencies, city health officials, civic organizations, the media, and other groups.

The Five-Day Plan is not a religious program. That is to say, no doctrine, creed, or dogma of any nature is given. Naturally, if you are religious, you are encouraged to seek divine aid. Whatever your preference, the Five-Day Plan insists on complete withdrawal. No tapering off. The author of this book attended this clinic for five evenings. It worked.

The Five-Day Plan has been successful with youth groups, factory employees, and the blind. In Norway and the Philippines it is the government-supported program. Japanese health agencies have endorsed it; a pocket-sized book of the concepts is sold by the hundreds of thousands in the streets of Japan. The American Broadcasting Company prepared a series of half-hour films of the Five-Day Plan; these films were aired several times in San Francisco, Miami, Denver, Chicago, and many other cities throughout the United States, as well as in Toronto, Canada. Many radio stations and independent television stations have offered this plan on an evening or daytime basis. Some three thousand people turned out for a first stop smoking seminar in Mexico City, and over two thousand participated in Torino, Italy.

Some Helpful Hospitals

In the United States, the Five-Day Plan is associated with many major hospitals. A few of them are listed here:

St. Helena Hospital
Deer Park, California 94576

Glendale Adventist Medical Center
1509 Wilson Terrace
Glendale, California 91206

Loma Linda University Medical Center
Loma Linda, California 92354

White Memorial Medical Center

1720 Brooklyn Avenue
Los Angeles, California 90033

Feather River Hospital
5974 Pentz Road
Paradise, California 95969

Boulder Memorial Hospital
311 Mapleton Avenue
Boulder, Colorado 80302

Porter's Memorial Hospital
2525 South Downing
Denver, Colorado 80210

Florida Hospital
601 East Rollins Street
Orlando, Florida 32803

Hinsdale Sanitarium and Hospital
120 North Oak Street
Hinsdale, Illinois 60521

Shawnee Medical Center
74th and Grandview
Shawnee Mission, Kansas 66201

Washington Adventist Hospital
Takoma Park, Maryland 20012

New England Memorial Hospital
5 Woodland Road
Stoneham, Massachusetts 02180

Kettering Medical Center
Kettering, Ohio 45429

Portland Adventist Medical Center
10123 Southeast Market Street
Portland, Oregon 97216

Madison Hospital
500 Hospital Drive
Madison, Tennessee 37115

Huguley Memorial Hospital
P.O. Box 6337
Fort Worth, Texas 76115

Walla Walla General Hospital
Walla Walla, Washington 99362

Other Useful Addresses

Ask about programs and free kits or literature on smoking from the following organizations:

Office on Smoking and Health
Rockville, Maryland 20857

American Cancer Society, Inc.
National Headquarters
777 Third Avenue
New York, New York 10017

American Lung Association
1740 Broadway
New York, New York 10019

Department of Health Education
Porter Memorial Hospital
2525 South Downing
Denver, Colorado 80210

American Heart Association
5415 Maple
Dallas, Texas 75235

The Five-Day Plan
6840 Eastern Avenue, N.W.
Washington, D.C. 20012

Narcotics Education, Inc.
6830 Laurel Street, N.W.
Washington, D.C. 20012

CHAPTER FIVE

Hypnosis and "B.T."

Around thirty million Americans have given up cigarettes. Some have done it in very unusual ways. Other people preferred various therapies or paid for the commercial stop smoking clinics. There is a theory behind paying anywhere from $50 to $500 for such help: when you lay your own (or your parents') dollars on the line for a program, you will probably attend all of the sessions. A free clinic doesn't demand any investment on your part. Therefore, smokers may choose not to come every time. But plunking down your hard-earned savings from a summer job is great motivation to attend the entire program of a clinic.

Remember that not one of the methods for quitting is a sure thing. Some of them work only for some people. Even spending good cash doesn't guarantee a foolproof cure. It is also true that you may not require any of these programs right now.

But the need will increase at some point in your life.

In the next pages we will look into the many possibilities available to help you shed the smoking habit. You will hear about some new ideas in psychology and acquire a better understanding of older psychological theories that work.

Getting Yourself Hypnotized

You enter a small, quiet office. On a desk are a calendar, a clock, a blotter. You see a paper basket; a green plant stands in the corner. The hypnotist is a tall, blonde woman in her thirties. She sits across from you in a straight chair. She offers you a chair; you can recline on it. You're very comfortable and not at all nervous. You talked to her at length the day before. You know what will happen.

There's no reason to be freaked out. Clinical hypnosis has nothing to do with the kind presented on television, on the stage, or in novels.

No one makes you go into a deep sleep or hypnotizes you to act silly. In fact, the hypnotist cannot make you do anything against your will. She needs your cooperation at all times. You have control over your actions.

The young woman is highly trained. She attended the American College of Clinical Hypnosis in Philadelphia, Pennsylvania. She isn't a physician or a psychiatrist; she is a clinical hypnotist.

The hypnotist's voice is quiet and soothing. She asks you about the last cigarette you had. You remember it, and you talk about it. The heat in your mouth. The burning throat. The pain in your lungs as you inhaled. The weight on your chest. Your heart pumping fast.

"But now you're well," the hypnotist says. "You're calm. And you're comfortable, right?"

"Right."

"Yes, settle back. Relax your legs. Relax your toes. And your ankles, too. Tense them for a second, and then let go. Breathe deeply, deeply. Close your eyes. Relax your toes. How does it feel?"

"Good."

"Concentrate on relaxing. Your toes, your ankles, your legs. Your arms, too. Let go. Let go. Breathe deeply." The hypnotist's voice is soft, serene, a little dull, almost drowsy, as if she were going to sleep. "Fine. Relax. Toes. Ankles. Legs. Arms."

She speaks for another five minutes—or is it ten? It is difficult to keep track of time. Gradually, you begin to feel light-headed; the sensation has been compared to floating. It is still possible to open your eyes, to see the hypnotist. If the phone rang, you would hear it shrill through the room.

Yet you're already in a trance.

At this stage, everything depends on whether you really want to quit smoking. If you've made up your mind to give up cigarettes—and real motivations are needed for this step—you can get some good help now.

Hypnosis makes smokers susceptible to dropping the habit. You can be influenced while you are in a trance. The hypnotist does the most important work during the next ten to twenty minutes.

"Tell me about your last cigarette. Do you remember how it tasted?"

"Yes, I do."

"How did it taste?"

"Hot and bitter."

"That's all?"

"No, it burned my lungs. Ton of weight on my chest. . . ."

"It wasn't very good, was it?" suggests the hypnotist. "And now? No more desire to smoke cigarettes, right?"

"No more. I'm through with them. . . ."

"You can quit now, you no longer want cigarettes. Tobacco actually turns you off."

"Sure does. Tobacco is a bummer."

"You won't even become irritable without cigarettes, right? In fact, you'll be cheerful. You're winning a battle against a habit. You've quit, quit!"

There are approximately 15,000 persons in the United States who are qualified hypnotists. Some of them are medical doctors, psychiatrists, and psychologists. Others, like the actual hypnotist described above, were trained for six months or longer.

The approach to your smoking problem may differ from hypnotist to hypnotist. Dr. William Nemon, a well-known expert, whispers to his patients, "Tobacco is poison to your body. . . . You need your body to live. . . . You can't allow more poisoning of your body." Dr. Herbert Spiegel, an East Coast leader in the field, puts you into a mild trance, and then says, "I need my body to live. I owe my body this respect. . . . " Lester Palmer, a Colorado hypnotist, takes the positive approach: "You enjoy being a nonsmoker. . . . It is much better to be a nonsmoker. . . . "

Can everyone be hypnotized?

Retarded people and very analytical people make poor subjects. "Hypnosis is a game you play with your own imagination," says one specialist. "People must be able to relax and go with it in order for hypnosis to work."

Experts also generally agree that the system doesn't work for a young person who is easily distracted. You must be able to concentrate, to pay attention. About 80 percent of the population can be hypnotized. For some people, of course, it takes longer to reach a trancelike state. Others can do it within minutes.

The number of sessions a person needs to quit smoking varies. Some specialists, like those of the American Clinic, Inc. (which you can find in twenty cities, with headquarters in Campbell, California 95008), recommend at least seven sessions of about one hour each. The program costs around $300. Other experts say that one hour can be enough. Dr. Herbert Spiegel, perhaps the best known clinical hypnotist in America, has achieved success in just forty-five minutes. The time is spent mostly on teaching you to use self-hypnosis which ensures long-lasting results.

Self-hypnosis

Self-hynosis is a safe method, recommended by many stop smoking experts. Before you do self-hynosis, however, discuss it with your family doctor.

You learn to relax so well that you can put yourself into a light trance. At that point, you give yourself instruction to quit smoking cigarettes. You need a quiet room and fifteen to thirty minutes of privacy for this.

First, make yourself comfortable, either lying down or sitting. The idea is to find a position, arms to the sides and legs uncrossed, that will cause the least amount of fidgeting.

Begin by taking a deep breath. Hold it for five seconds, then breathe normally for ten seconds. Take another deep breath, hold it for five seconds, and mentally spell *relax* while exhaling. On the *x*, close your eyes.

Now shift your attention to your feet. Imagine the muscles relaxing. Notice the tingling in your feet, especially on the bottom. Next, move to your calves and imagine them relaxing. Then move to your thighs, stomach, and so on, relaxing each set of muscles in turn.

Be sure to continue to your chin, cheeks, eyebrows, and the top of your head. You can shift your position at any time. Just take a slow, deep breath and return to where you left off.

Your breathing has now slowed. Feel the rise and fall of your chest. Each time you exhale, tell yourself you are going deeper and deeper into a trancelike feeling. Do this several times. Then, on every other breath, begin to count backward from five to one, telling yourself that each number is increasing the relaxed feeling.

At the count of one, you will be in a light state of hypnosis. Now you'll be able to talk yourself into giving up cigarettes.

How about the trance? How do you come out of it? No one ever gets stuck in this special state. You may become sleepy and then wake up refreshed. Most people compare this light trance to intense meditation. If you meditate, you know you can terminate it any time you want to.

Some hypnotists let their clients count from one to five. Do it slowly, and at the count of five, open your eyes. You will then be wide awake, feeling fine and in perfect health.

You can use self-hypnosis several times a day or every time you crave a cigarette. Some clinics suggest at least ten or more self-hypnosis sessions a day. But these sessions need not last more than twenty seconds to a minute.

Experts agree that self-hypnosis has great advantages. It allows you to get involved with yourself. You begin to take responsibility for your own actions. You no longer depend on a therapist.

Self-hypnosis can only be effective against the weed if you really make up your mind to stop smoking. Hypnosis won't do any good unless you actually want to kick the habit. One psychologist explains it this way: "If your smoking enjoyment is stronger than your wish to quit, you will be ignoring your own suggestion to quit."

You should also know that ethical hypnotists never promise you 100 percent success; not every person can stop through this method. It requires your cooperation with the therapist. Even more important, hypnosis wears off. One of the most interesting studies was made by Dr. G. Grayson of San Francisco. At the International Conference on Lung Diseases, Dr. Grayson reported the results of a four-week clinic with eight hypnosis sessions.

There were 233 smokers. Of the 233, only 180 quit cigarettes for up to ten months. Just 73 persons of the original 233 were cured up to two years or longer.

What does this prove? "The crux of success really depends on the individual's true desire to stop," says Dr. Grayson. "Some people really don't want to quit. They ask for hypnosis when in fact they want something else, like help to get over loneliness, for instance. Asking for hypnosis is then merely a cover for the person's real needs."

It has also been found that your motivation to quit must be clear to you. Your reason has to be more than "My folks told me to quit" or "My girl friend says she'll love me better." What's more, self-hypnosis is the key, and anyone who is serious about the method had better learn it.

All in all, however, clinical hypnosis need not scare you. It is safe, and it has proven useful in many cases.

If you want to try this method, find a good hypnotist by calling your state medical society for names of physicians or psychiatrists who use hypnosis. If you live in a large community, check the yellow pages of the phone book under "Psychologists." One final possibility: check under "Hypnotists." When you call someone, ask if the person belongs to the American Society of Clinical Hypnosis, or has a diploma from the American College of Clinical Hypnosis. Both are respectable organizations.

Help from Behavior Therapy

Behavior therapy is a popular term right now. It means the process of changing behavior patterns, for instance, in regard to smoking. The change, or modification, can often be achieved in a few hours with a therapist. B.T. can involve either a psychiatrist or a psychologist. Various people in the physical or mental health fields, such as nurses, often offer an inexpensive program, too. In the end, however, it's up to the client to follow through.

B.T. consists of a few easy steps:

1. You decide what behavior you want to change. In this case, it's smoking.
2. With the help of the therapist, you find out why you smoke and why you want to quit.
3. You make up your mind that you will quit.

Thinking things out is one of the musts for success in this method. The Five-Day Plan developers, for instance, suggest that you say these things to yourself:

● Smoking is basically a selfish habit, a habit that gratifies personal desires.
● There was no good reason to start smoking. I began only because of social pressures.
● It's a foolish habit; many people smoke despite the danger of sickness.

One of the greatest modern researchers in the field of behavior therapy is Dr. David Premack, a Santa Barbara, California, psychologist after whom "the Premack principle" has been named. In brief, it works like this. You write down five statements against smoking and five statements on why you want to quit. The statements are written on index cards which you post around your room, in the bathroom, and on your most-used books. You can even place a card on top of your television set. This way, you can look at the list all the time. Some antismoking statements are:

1. Smoking is a disgusting habit.
2. My smoking makes me feel sick about myself.
3. I'm that much closer to cancer by smoking each day.
4. I'm so ashamed that I can't or won't stop.
5. I feel terrible that my sister (brother) might pick up my habit.

Five Premack pro-quitting statements are:

1. Each minute I don't smoke, my lungs grow clearer.
2. Food will taste so much better.
3. Everyone will be proud of me when I quit.
4. Quitting will put years on my life.

> 5.   Good-bye cigarettes, good-bye cough, good-bye sore throats.

In a few days, you should be brainwashed enough to really end the habit.

A good therapist will tailor the program for different kinds of smokers. An adult smoker must learn to break the habit chain. A young person who smokes mostly to impress others could find other ways to make an impression on his or her peers.

B.T. merely means unlearning one pattern (like smoking) and learning a new one.

Behavior modification actually started long ago. It began with Ivan Pavlov, the great Russian physician who was born in 1849 and received a Nobel Prize for his work in 1904. Dr. Pavlov became famous for his experiments with a dog. At the sound of a bell he would feed meat to the dog. After a while, the animal would salivate at the bell's ringing alone. Dr. Pavlov called this the conditioned reflex. He theorized that such a response actually applies not only to animals but to people as well.

Specifically, a young smoker may condition herself or himself to light a cigarette in a school yard at the sight of other girls or boys who are smoking. A young smoker may condition herself or himself to hunger for a cigarette at a party where everyone drinks beer. If you attend such beer parties several nights a week, you condition yourself to smoke each time until it becomes a hard to break habit.

What do the B.T. specialists suggest?

Like the Five-Day Plan organizers, they help you avoid the Pavlovian stimuli that cause you to smoke. You don't go to the school yard where the other smoking students assemble. (And you ignore the peer pressure by telling them that you've decided to breathe fresh air instead of tobacco smoke.) You shun the parties where everyone guzzles booze and fills the ashtrays with stubs. In fact, behavior therapists advise that you dispose of ashtrays and matches. If you smoke at a certain desk in your home, now do your studying at another desk.

Unlearning a habit is not easy, but it can be done. You just rearrange your life to achieve control over your behavior. After a few weeks, it is you who has attained the goal. The therapist has long ago become unnecessary. It's all do-it-yourself from now on.

Psychologists suggest that quitters should promise themselves special rewards. If you stay off the weed for two full weeks, promise to buy yourself the jacket, sweater, or dress you've long wanted. Treat a friend to an expensive show.

It has been found that behavior therapy does not always have a long-range effect. Some people drift back to their old ways when there is sudden tension or anxiety. However, they've made a start at quitting, and this often leads to a second try that turns out to be a success.

Aversion Therapy

Aversion therapy is classed among the behavior therapies.

Also known as aversive conditioning, the technique attempts to couple unwanted behavior (like smoking) with an unpleasant or painful experience. Aversion therapy can involve electrical shocks: you get a jolt as soon as you pick up a cigarette or the instant you inhale smoke. This kind of therapy works on the punishment principle. One specialist explains it this way: "The subconscious responds basically to pain and pleasure. If we remove all the pleasure from a habit and replace it with discomfort (pain), the subconscious will not be motivated to continue the habit."

The discomfort or pain can be mild, such as someone snapping a rubber band against your wrist as you pick up your cigarette. Inhaling the stink of lighted tobacco and very rapid smoking have both been used. The therapist makes you smoke too much and too fast so that you become sick to your stomach, a condition you remember later when you want to reach for another smoke. Another system has a machine blowing smoke into your face. Your eyes start to water, your nose gets irritated, and you cough.

Still one more aversion technique is having the person smoke in a small, closed space that is hot and dry. The idea here is that you will find the situation unpleasant. The room becomes filled with dense smoke, and you are unable to breathe in comfort.

Dr. Bedford's Experiments

One of the aversion therapy pioneers is Dr. Stewart Bedford, a Chico, California, psychologist and lecturer. His own interest in smoking cessation was stirred up when he had to work with groups of eight to twelve people.

"These group therapy sessions, or marathon workshops, last from two to thirty hours," Dr. Bedford explains. "I got tired of sitting for long periods in a smoke-filled room. So I decided to ban smoking. People could indulge, but they had to leave, one at a time, and do their thing on a covered patio attached to my office."

When he studied the literature in the specialized aversion field, Dr. Bedford read about the smoking chamber.

After much thought and a period at the drawing board, the psychologist came up with the idea of a mock-up lung large enough for one person to sit in. He built an egg-shaped contraption with a cover that enclosed the individual. The device had a wire frame and was covered with asbestos and thick paper. Inside there was a switch so that the patient could control the light.

The psychologist placed this object in the smoking area and suggested that the cigarette smokers

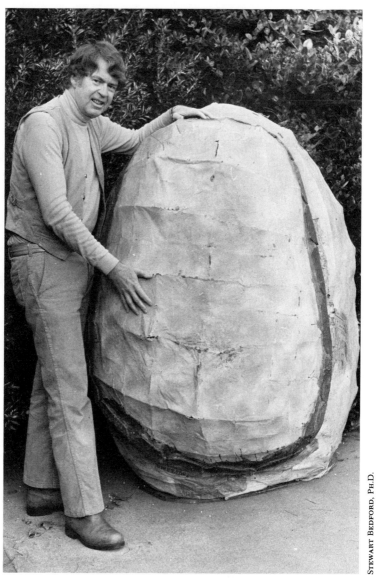

Dr. Stewart Bedford and his smoking chamber.

in the group use this whenever they wanted to take their nicotine break. Dr. Bedford also suggested that the smokers talk to the rest of the people about their experiences in the "lung monster."

One day someone suggested that smokers carry on an imaginary conversation between their own lungs and their brains. What would their lungs say to their brains if lungs could speak for themselves?

The idea of the "talking lung" sounded a little nutty at first. However, the smokers thought it was a good idea and agreed to try it. Would the lungs complain to the smokers' heads and cause the brains to tell the smokers to quit? Not so. The lungs did complain. The brains did tell the cigarette addicts to stop, but the smokers enjoyed the whole procedure and kept right on puffing away.

The doctor went back to the drawing board. Eventually success was achieved. Dr. Bedford incorporated the lung monster with individual psychological therapy. The psychologist and most of his colleagues combine aversion systems with counseling. Like other experts, the Californian found that the techniques can only help if the smokers understand why they smoke.

Rapid Smoking

Some of the practitioners in the field also use other techniques. They make smokers inhale rapidly, for instance, or the addicted adults are invited to puff one cigarette after another. After about five minutes, the people are pretty sick of even their favorite brand. In fact, the smokers cannot tolerate one more tobacco cloud.

This is known as the satiation system. It means that you're more than satisfied. What's more, you're nauseated.

At one big commercial center (which demands $450 for this experience) the patient is almost always an adult. A businessman enrolled in one of these clinics. He was made to step into a sort of telephone booth. According to him, "The therapist stood at the door, wearing an army surplus gas mask! She told me to puff as fast as I could." The executive soon found himself choking. The lighted butt was so hot that it felt as if his tongue were afire.

When the businessman puffed one more cigarette inside the booth, he became extremely dizzy. He hoped that the ordeal was over, but it wasn't.

He describes what happened next: "After ten drags, I was so dizzy that I could barely keep myself sitting upright on the chair. The therapist told me to put the cigarette out and light another. Soon my hands, feet, and legs felt numb and damp. In addition, I couldn't think straight."

As the man started the third cigarette, the therapist asked if his stomach was upset. It wasn't. About halfway through, though, the poor fellow began to belch and taste stomach bile backing up into his throat.

Almost at the end of the smoke, the man's neck and forehead suddenly felt cold and clammy. The therapist in the gas mask said that his face had taken on an ashen hue. The executive remembers it this way: "Shaking, I could not walk straight as I emerged from the booth. I felt totally disoriented. If someone had asked me to solve two plus two, it probably would have taken a minute or so to figure out the answer.

"The next fellow practically fainted after the first cigarette and had to be led to a window for some fresh air and a break. At the beginning of the third cigarette, he got a sick stomach. A third man became sick in the middle of the second cigarette."

Physicians warn that a person must get a good medical checkup before trying this technique. One of the warnings comes from Dr. David P.L. Sachs. He monitored twenty-four healthy young men while at the Stanford Medical School. The test group was made to take a puff every six seconds. The gases in the cigarettes cut sharply into the young people's blood oxygen levels. One of the smokers experienced an arterial oxygen drop so severe that it would have killed someone with heart disease, says the doctor. "Luckily, the young men were all healthy." Dr. Sachs concludes, "Rapid smoking should only be risked after a pulmonary lung function test and an EKG (heart test)."

CHAPTER SIX

A Mix of Programs for Big (and Little) Spenders

Zap! Zap! Zap!

Of all the stop smoking clinics, the Schick Centers might well be the most fascinating.

The firm explains its theories this way: "During the Schick program, pleasurable links that formed habits fade away gradually by first removing the pleasure associated with the habit. As the client goes through the motions of smoking, he develops an increasing boredom and then distaste for these substances as they cease to provide pleasure or relaxation. In addition, the cigarette becomes linked to discomfort."

Apart from using electrical impulses, the system also employs the "rapid smoking" and "satiation" smoking chamber about which you read in the previous chapter. The "therapists," who don't need a degree in medicine or psychology, back these tactics with lectures on the danger of cigarettes to your health. Sessions last for one hour and go on for five days. After that the patient need only return once a week for eight weeks to listen to lectures and see films.

The numerous Schick offices are scattered throughout the western and southern United States. According to government reports, the aversion techniques "have largely failed to help people quit smoking. . . . " Schick's own national figures look better. Officials say that after one year, 53 percent of the patients were off cigarettes.

The Black Box

Treatment generally takes place in a room with several small booths. Each booth has two straight chairs, two one-foot-square low tables, and a curtain across its door. Before you is an ashtray. The floor is strewn with ashes and hundreds of half-smoked, stale butts. On the table next to the other chair you see a black box with switches, dials, and wires. The box becomes known as the "shock box" during the week.

Attached to the box are two electrical leads that terminate at two large rivets mounted on a rubber belt. When the belt is wrapped around your wrist, a button is pressed on the black box. You suddenly feel an irritating electrical shock. The intensity can be increased by turning a dial on the box. For safety, the machine is designed to produce a current low enough not to be dangerous. But the jolt of electricity is distressing.

Many people have described the Schick system as the most unpleasant method of quitting smoking. The process starts with your being hooked up to the box by means of an electrode. A little cold cream is dabbed in the rivets to make contact with your skin. You are then told how the machine works. The therapist sits behind you with a finger on the button of the shock box.

Now comes the treatment. You are asked to light a cigarette from one of the three packs lying on the table before you. Three different types of cigarettes are offered—a nonfilter, menthol, and filter.

The therapist says, "Do not inhale. Think of the cigarette as you draw the smoke in and blow it out. Lay the cigarette down after each puff and lean back. Okay, now go ahead. Smoke!"

As you hold the burning match to your cigarette, you feel a series of shocks on your wrist. The electricity ceases as soon as you put the cigarette down.

One patient explains what happens next: "I reached again for my cigarette. And zap! Zap! Zap! The shocks start all over!" This goes on until you've smoked about half of the weed. You're next asked to pick up a sample from two other brands. Each puff is being properly punished with electrical charges.

Sometimes, the jolt comes when you inhale. At other times, it comes as you reach for the cigarette.

The shock treatment lasts about an hour. The next day, you come back for more. The rest of the aversion clinic consists of the patient puffing away in a Schick booth. The therapist sometimes stands by in a gas mask.

Lectures on the toxic substances in cigarettes and some general advice round out the program.

SmokEnders

Government workers recently took part in a federally sponsored stop smoking clinic.

The people were employed by the U. S. Public Health Service, a division of the Department of Health, Education and Welfare. PHS chose SmokEnders to conduct its program for the agency's employees. More than 175 persons took part. About 135 people stopped smoking during the eight-week program.

SmokEnders is one of the largest and most successful smoke cessation programs of its kind in the country. It has many chapters from coast to coast and in Canada. In fact, you will find a chapter in every major city.

The organization has not only worked with Uncle Sam's employees, like those of HEW, but also with some hospitals, colleges, and large corporations. The clinics often take place at hotels or motels.

At least 100,000 people have quit since Smok-Enders started in 1969. Among the quitters were a number of thirteen-year-olds who had smoked their first cigarettes at the age of eight. Most of the clients are in their twenties or older.

The program consists of eight weekly meetings —two hours per session—after school or work hours.

For the first five weeks, the moderators insist that you continue to smoke. In fact, you can puff away as much as you like until the program develops your motivation to call it quits and to change your attitude. By means of behavior therapy, you

Jacquelyn Rogers warns young people that they waste money by smoking.

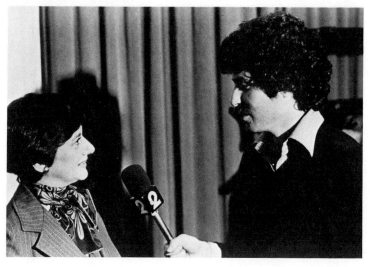

JACQUELYN ROGERS—SMOKENDERS

will slowly steer toward the big moment when you can quit.

At SmokEnders this takes five weeks.

In fact, you are somewhat prepared for cut-off day.

It is the crucial day for the participants. After that, there are only three more sessions.

A SmokEnders executive explains the concept. "This is no medical program. We do not dispense drugs or medical advice. We employ no scare tactics, hypnosis, sermonizing, or pressure. We point no fingers, do no shouting, call no names. We teach."

SmokEnders' advertising hits hard. "Last year, we freed 30,000 slaves!" reads one headline. Another proclaims, "You will stop smoking on June 2nd!"

The ads overcome objections such as these:

> "But I smoke three packs a day." (It doesn't matter. Whether you smoke three cigarettes or three packs a day, you may be equally addicted. And you can quit just as easily.)
> "But I don't have any willpower." (It doesn't matter. All you need is enough willpower to come to our meetings.)

The it's-a-cinch idea is used by the speakers too; all of them are former smokers who convince you that you will stop painlessly, calmly, comfortably.

The smokers' standard defenses are hit in the first session:

> "I enjoy smoking." (No, you do it because it's addictive and you're uncomfortable without a cigarette, so when you get one, it relieves your discomfort and you have been taught to label it "enjoyment.")
> "If I quit, I'll get fat." (There are weight controls built into the SmokEnders plan.)
> "I concentrate better with a cigarette." (Smoking actually cuts your mental capacity.)
> "I need cigarettes to relax and stay calm." (Cigarette smoke is a stimulant and jangles the nerves.)

The speaker also adds to your reasons why you should stop. At the typical clinic you will be told that smokers have 23 percent poorer memories than nonsmokers. Each cigarette takes five and a half minutes off a smoker's life. Smokers have a 200 percent better chance of dying than nonsmokers in the same age group.

Like many programs, SmokEnders wisely reminds you of how smoking hits you in the pocket. The group leader tells you that cigarette prices are rising. A pack will soon cost a dollar. Even if you only buy one pack a day (which is typical for teenage smokers), you will spend almost $400 a year.

SmokEnders also emphasizes the high cost of cigarettes in its junior programs. In fact, the founder herself wisely told a large group of teenagers:

> It is very expensive to smoke, especially for young people on allowances. Ask your friends to consider the cost of smoking: daily, weekly, monthly, yearly, and over a lifetime. The total spent at any one point could provide them with many of the luxuries and pleasures which may not be realized otherwise. Ask your friends to translate those dollars into gas money, records, or whatever they're into. We demonstrate that a person of eighteen who smokes a pack and a half a day will have spent enough in ten years to have bought a new Corvette!

SmokEnders was started in 1969 by Jacquelyn Rogers, a New Jersey mother who was herself addicted for twenty-two years. As the wife of Dr. Jon Rogers, a dentist, she knew well enough that she shouldn't ruin her gums, teeth, throat, and lungs. After some solid research, Jackie worked up a plan to stop smoking herself. She picked as cut-off day her wedding anniversary. Afterward, as a reward, the couple went to Vermont on a skiing vacation.

The Jackie Rogers method relies on these steps:

- Deciding why you want to stop (motivation).
- Being determined to stop (behavior modification).

- Doing it together with others (group dynamics).
- Gradual withdrawal.
- Fighting withdrawal symptoms (with fruit juice).
- Substituting activities (waterskiing, jogging, and so forth).

Instead of the Five-Day Plan slogan, "I choose not to smoke," the SmokEnder system says, "I don't smoke anymore."

Does it really succeed? One young listener gives his impression of that first SmokEnders get-together. "It may well work. But I was left with one fact. It's still up to me to quit. No one can do it for me."

Can You Stop with Special Drugs?

The world's powerful drug industry has long marketed special products for smokers.

You can buy pills of all kinds without prescription. There is also an anticigarette chewing gum with a mint flavor. In some foreign countries—Sweden, for example—pharmaceuticals are injected into the smoker's body.

The Swedes favor lobeline, a nicotine substitute. In the United States, lobeline has been available in drugstores under brand names such as Bantron, Nikoban, and others. Lobeline is supposed to help you get over the withdrawal symptoms after quitting. The substitute for nicotine in your system may help lessen the craving for actual cigarettes. Such a substitute cannot stop you from buying another carton of your favorite brand. In fact, surveys show that many smokers soon go back to their normal cigarette consumption.

Some antismoking products contain a tranquilizer to calm you down. Certain pharmaceuticals make cigarettes taste so bad that you may stop smoking for a while. One such product, Deter, is sold in small bottles. You tap a few drops onto the back of your tongue. Now you're protected against the habit for about two hours. As long as you don't touch a cigarette, you will hardly be aware of Deter in your mouth, except that it freshens your breath. Deter is not a stimulant or a tranquilizer. You can eat or drink, drive a car, attend school, do whatever you like. The only thing that will give you a hard time is smoking. A Deter brochure tells what happens: "The instant your willpower fails you and you light up, Deter goes to work. We promise you unconditionally that your first puff will taste so terrible—so downright awful—that you won't want a second puff!"

Apart from drugs, a few other gimmicks have been tried by smokers. Some firms sell special filters that reduce cigarette tars and nicotine. The smoker supposedly gets used to lower and lower levels of these poisons. One day, so the theory goes, he or she need not smoke at all. There is nothing wrong with this idea, except that it only works for the person who smokes occasionally.

Switching Instead of Stopping

Some people decide that they need not stop at all. How about switching to a low tar, filter cigarette? It is true that modern cigarette filters trap much of the tar and nicotine that damage human beings. The tar content of the average cigarette is now 50 percent lower than it was before you were born, and 30 percent lower than it was ten years ago. In addition, cigarette companies now use more tobacco stems and other discards; this reduces the tars still further. You can now get some brands that contain only 0.5 milligrams of tar per cigarette. The nicotine level of some new filter cigarettes can be as low as 0.05 milligrams.

A Safe Cigarette

The invention and heavy use of the filter made some public health officials hope that the lung cancer rate would go down. No such thing happened, however. Filter users were still developing this disease four times more often than nonsmokers. Year after year, despite the soaring use of "hifi" (high filtration), the lung disease figures stayed on the same level.

Medical researchers were at first baffled. How could this be? The tars and nicotine had been cut. Gradually, some interesting facts came to light:

- According to a Harvard University study, the filter smokers inhaled more deeply and held smoke longer in their lungs.
- The low tar cigarettes allowed just as much or more of the deadly carbon monoxide and other gases to reach the lungs.
- The filter cigarettes gave less tobacco and fewer toxic tars and nicotine poisons. True addicts, who continued to crave strong tobacco, now had to smoke twice as much to meet the nicotine need. All kinds of tobacco substitutes—like tea or

No safe cigarette exists.

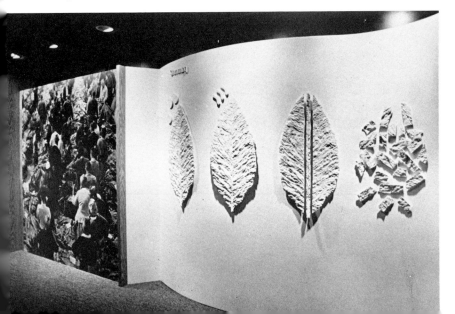

cabbage leaves and even seaweed—brought few steady customers. People went back to their double ration of filters.

Is there such a thing as a "safe" cigarette? Experts don't think so. After checking for years into the "safety" of the low tar, low nicotine smoke, Jacquelyn Rogers of SmokEnders blasted the cigarette makers in no uncertain terms.

Listen to her. "The public is being ripped off," she warns. "There can never be a safe material to inhale into our lungs in the smoky state. It doesn't matter if it is orange rinds; if it's burning and smoking and you inhale it, you're causing yourself problems. . . ."

In an equally serious vein, Dr. Stanley Schachter of Columbia University warned his colleagues that "low tar brands are now hooking millions of teenagers. . . ."

The only safe thing to do is quit. What is it like to quit? How about those first few days? What happens after two weeks?

The next chapter tells you all.

CHAPTER SEVEN

Quitting Forever

Fighting Withdrawal Symptoms

During the day, the man was in torment. During the night, he had trouble sleeping. He gasped at times. He kept thinking of cigarettes. He was groggy when he awoke. His first impulse was to reach for a cigarette. But there was none. He had quit smoking.

At first, he thought he couldn't get through the working day. He felt on edge, irritated, helpless, a changed person. He found it difficult to concentrate, to do his job. In business for himself, he had wisely changed the location of his work area, where he had smoked for so many years. Instead of the basement, he now earned his living on the first floor of his home.

In the afternoon, his temples throbbed. He had a dull headache. Every few minutes, he felt a

129

severe craving for a smoke. He fought the craving, and it went away. An hour later, the urge returned and was even stronger. It affected the juices in his mouth. The thought of tobacco made his mouth water as if for food.

When he talked to people, he didn't know what to do with his hands. He had used his right hand for flicking ashes during three decades. Now he couldn't. At first, he almost automatically reached into the pocket where he had kept his cigarettes for so many years.

He alternately felt tired or nervous. At other times, he was light-headed or dizzy. There was always this terrible craving, this lusting after a smoke. Just one smoke! The need pursued him into his sleep; he was actually puffing away in a dream. He smoked a whole pack in a few minutes. Then he *ate* a pack. The bitter, nauseating taste awoke him. He felt cranky all day. These are an adult chain smoker's withdrawal symptoms, the author's symptoms when he quit smoking.

Young people have it easier. Most of you haven't smoked for very long or very much.

Breaking off therefore poses less of a problem. It's no big deal.

The withdrawal symptoms, if any, will be slight.

Why the Discomforts Decrease

Let's say you are now seventeen years old. You sneaked your first cigarette at the age of twelve. You eventually worked up to one pack a day. You were on the way to becoming a two-pack smoker when you figured you'd better quit. You did, two days ago.

Since you were a real smoker, you must expect some tobacco withdrawal symptoms. As one young former chain puffer put it, "I was at first a little lost. Each time I wanted a cigarette but couldn't have one, my body rebelled a little. It was saying, 'Where is that nicotine?' But I had no answer."

Physiologically, your craving stems from the sudden absence of nicotine in your bloodstream. Even a young body can get used to nicotine, provided the person smokes one or more packs a day for six months or longer. When you quit, the deprivation can lower your blood pressure. The lack of nicotine also decreases the sugar level in your liver.

These withdrawal symptoms may increase during the second and third days. The body must adjust to the new conditions. For the heavy smoker, this may take a week or longer.

You can help speed up the process. There are some proven devices. Psychologically, you can fight the cravings this way: Look at a watch, see the seconds tick by, and say to yourself, "I choose not to smoke for two minutes." At the end of that period, the craving will be gone. You will be free of it until the next onset, minutes or hours later, depending on how long and how much you smoked. For the heavy consumers, the cravings come in predictable cycles, but these cycles will subside.

Avoid the places where you used to smoke. If you did it while studying at a certain table, study elsewhere now. If you lit up during a certain television program, go to a movie instead. In any case, keep busy. This way the craving won't surface as often.

Physically, withdrawal symptoms can be fought by means of the time-proven methods of the Five-Day Plan.

1. This is the time really to enjoy luxury. Take a warm bath two or three times a day for fifteen to twenty minutes. Just relax. If you feel you cannot stand not smoking any longer, hop right back into the tub, or the shower. It's pretty hard to smoke in a shower.

2. Drink six to eight glasses of water or juice between meals. The more liquids you can down, the quicker the nicotine is flushed out of your body. Swallowing fluids also satisfies the tickling and soothes the irritation in the throat. The motions and activity of getting the beverage and the process of drinking it satisfy the demand to use your hands.

3. Get adequate rest during these five days, eat complete meals at regular times, and pick a reasonable time to go to bed (eight hours of sleep won't hurt you).

4. After meals, go outside, walk, and breathe deeply for fifteen to thirty minutes. Do not sit in your favorite chair after eating. Exercise is a great way to relax, to work off tensions and work out worries. Try a twenty-minute walk after dinner instead of smoking an after-dinner cigarette. Walking helps you digest your food and fills your lungs with fresh air instead of smoke. Take a friend along.

5. Do not drink alcohol, tea, coffee, or cola beverages. Try to avoid all sedatives and stimulants, in order to build up a buffer against nervous tension as quickly as possible.

In some of the clinics, the directors also recommend that you rub yourself hard with a washcloth. They call this "cold mitten friction." It works on your blood circulation and gets you going in the morning. You can use somewhat cooler water every day. Deep breathing has long been an accepted help for quitters. Whenever the urge to smoke strikes, take five or six deep breaths, inhale very deeply, and exhale completely. This satisfies the physical craving to activate your breathing muscles, pumps large quantities of oxygen into your system, and thus helps calm your nerves. Many public speakers and concert singers practice deep breathing to relax them before a performance.

Dr. McFarland and other experts agree that the

smoking urge can remain strong during the first three days of withdrawal. Then the cravings weaken. At the end of five to seven days, you will be free of them. (For someone who only smoked one or two cigarettes a day, one day is probably enough.)

Drinking fluids will help clear your system. I recommend orange juice most of all; it helped me a great deal. You may notice you are thirstier than usual and perspire and urinate more than usual. To accelerate the flushing of your system, be sure to drink at least six glasses of water every day. Most people are so thirsty that they needn't be reminded.

Finally, to balance your blood sugar, eat plenty of high-protein foods. The more protein in your system, the less fluctuations in sugar and nicotine intake can affect your blood sugar levels.

Juices and vitamin C flush out the nicotine. Sports help your oxygen intake. The deadly carbon monoxide will be gone after the first twenty-four hours. Within a week, the former chain smoker can concentrate again; the brain starts functioning better than before. Two months later, the cilia in the smoker's lungs will once more become normal.

Consider the Benefits

This may be a good moment to count your blessings.

By getting over the cigarette habit you have:

- Embarked on a health route with fewer colds, sore throats, or morning coughs. You've improved your ability to play your favorite sports well.
- Earned the respect of those who count.
- Improved your future social life. You will never again smell up the rooms of non-smokers (who often despise smokers), burn anyone's furniture or clothes, or leave ashes around.
- Chucked a habit that would become more deeply ingrained later and far more difficult to break.
- Begun to save money. (Some ex-smokers actually figure out their weekly savings on a special scorecard.)

Reward Yourself

The cigarette ads often play on the theme that you should smoke to reward yourself. How about turning this around? Why not treat yourself especially well after you have quit smoking? In fact, psychologists suggest that you should pamper yourself during the first few days. You have a right to feel proud.

Consider the words of Buddha: "Though one should conquer a thousand men a thousand times, he who conquers himself has the more glorious

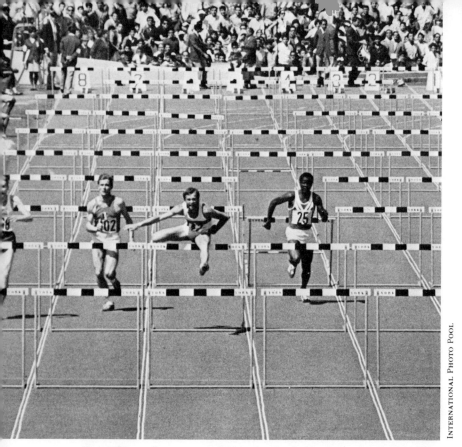

INTERNATIONAL PHOTO POOL

Benefits of not smoking include better running. No Olympic runner would touch a cigarette.

victory." The person who stops smoking deserves a better opinion of himself or herself. You're not a puppet now; you are your own person.

Will the Quitter Gain Weight?

The most experienced leaders in the stop smoking field claim that the former addict will find it challenging enough to stop smoking, especially if he or she was smoking one or more packs a day. Therefore, it would be unwise to make life more difficult by adding a diet on top of everything. There is an opposite view, however, that you should fast.

For a growing young person, a fast is hardly advisable, though, unless your doctor prescribes it for some reason.

Nutritionists, however, have gathered knowledge on certain food items that prove helpful during the first few days of quitting and on foods to avoid.

It makes sense, for instance, to stay clear of highly seasoned or peppery foods, Mexican dishes, spicy meats; these foods stimulate you to smoke. If you are eating at home, explain that you need simple, wholesome foods during your first week. Eat all the fresh vegetables, grains, and fruit you want. You can't overdo it in the fruit department. Many doctors recommend plenty of vitamin C in pill form, too, for extra amounts of vitamins. Particularly important is B complex. This is the vitamin to help your nicotine-deprived nerves. You can get B complex by taking a pill or by eating wheat germ. One or two tablespoons of brewer's yeast daily provide another good source.

There are several explanations for the ex-smoker's tendency to gain some weight. For one thing, the nervousness of the first few days without a cigarette leads to kitchen prowling. The empty hand reaches for a snack. What is more, an improved sense of smell makes your food more appealing. The taste buds suddenly work again.

Some ex-smokers may pick up a couple of pounds simply because they are healthier without cigarettes. Not smoking means you will have fewer heartbeats and a lower pulse rate, and so you will require fewer calories. The body gets more oxygen and functions more efficiently once smoke stops polluting your lungs. Digestion improves, and more food is used as fuel. Nonsmokers don't rush through their dinners as smokers do. They get more value from each meal. Your "new" body requires fewer calories, and yet you will probably be eating more. Even if you ate the same amount as you did when you smoked, you will gain some weight.

Specialists suggest that you do not worry about this. Enjoy yourself at the table. You may add a few pounds only for a period of a few months. Also, keep in mind that the weight-gain problem doesn't affect everyone, especially not the truly active, growing teenager.

In overweight, diet-conscious America, the fear of getting fat keeps many smokers puffing and causes some quitters to go back to cigarettes. Everyone has heard stories of ex-smokers getting fat.

The danger can be a real one, but nothing like the dangers of smoking. There are ways to give up cigarettes without gaining weight.

Apart from consuming a lot of juices, fruit, and

vegetables, stick to three meals a day. Start with a good breakfast. Many people skip breakfast and for the rest of the day try to catch up on nutrients.

The leaders of Five-Day Clinics, such as Dr. T. Kofoed, also warn that you should not substitute food for cigarettes. There is little point in giving up smoking and then eating too much. Smokers must watch their snacks. It is true that nibbling tempts those who have stopped smoking, and the American way of life encourages snacking.

Resist the temptation to grab handfuls of snack foods such as potato chips, peanuts, or candy instead of a cigarette. A snack is a great way to dodge that impulse to smoke. But make the snack light in calories and high in nutrition—fresh fruit, a hard-boiled egg, crisp vegetables, a cup of broth, or a glass of milk.

For Dieters

To be sure, some people get serious about their weight. Some girls worry if they put on even three extra pounds. This should cause no anxieties to ex-smokers.

To these diet-conscious people, one clinic offers these suggestions:

- Remove empty and refined calories from your diet as much as possible. (This includes white sugar and sweetened cereals. Go easy on ice cream, candy, cake, pies.) Eliminate or cut down drastically on all fats (bacon, oils, margarine, fattening salad dressings).

- Eat vegetables without additional amounts of butter or margarine; do not sweeten cereal; replace whole milk with low-fat milk or buttermilk.
- Avoid extra large portions and third servings.
- Get ahold of a calorie counter in the form of an inexpensive booklet.
- Exercise, too, is vital to the dieting ex-smoker.

"Just One Cigarette!"

The same behavioral scientists who specialize in the tobacco addiction problem also say that a former smoker must beware of just a single cigarette. "Why can't I have just one?" you may wonder. It seems that the one experimental cigarette gets you back to where you started. According to the psychologists, you become a backslider. (Others call this a "relapse.") This backsliding happens to be the greatest danger to the ex-smoker; compare the person's situation to that of the former teenage drinker who has stopped. If some pals offer him

more booze, he may once more turn into an alcoholic.

The Five-Day Plan leaders therefore point out
that you are not out of danger even after a week
or longer without cigarettes. Dr. Kofoed, who runs
the program in Denver, Colorado, makes these
sound suggestions:

- Stay clear of the smoking crowd during
  your school breaks. Avoid the area where
  they congregate.
- Avoid people who smoke in the school
  cafeteria. Don't sit at their tables.
- If anyone, even a friend or relative, offers
  you a cigarette, learn to say, "No, thanks.
  I have chosen to stop smoking." The person will not repeat the offer, and your
  words reinforce your own decision.
- If you find yourself under tension or in a
  pressure situation which would normally
  prompt a smoke, don't be tempted.
  Breathe deeply instead or take a short
  walk. This applies to a situation that may
  occur three months from now. (What if
  you should start smoking again? Well, it's
  not the end of the world. Just renew your
  struggle to quit; you will no doubt succeed the second time. Most people do.)
- Ignore anyone who claims that one cigarette won't hurt. It will. A backslider can
  wind up smoking more than before.

- Begin to consider yourself a nonsmoker. Look only to nonsmokers as your heroes. Forget about the famous television comic who chews Winstons, the movie cowboy who clouds up the camera lens with smoke, or the foolish crooner who may eventually lose his voice. Ask your parents what happened to some of the best-known movie idols of the past— Humphrey Bogart, for instance. Ask about the famous broadcaster Edward R. Murrow. Cigarette-associated cancer killed both of these men. Clark Gable, a heavy smoker, died of a heart attack.

- Throw out all your ashtrays and your packs of cigarettes. A New York City teenager quit after a severe addiction, but he made one mistake. He kept an open pack at home in his room. He would tempt himself by removing a cigarette and tapping it on his desk. He even stuck a cigarette playfully into his mouth. His parents told him he was playing with fire. The boy laughed. Two weeks later, he was back to thirty cigarettes a day, and he was again a loser at sports. This young man might benefit from the wise words of the Five-Day Plan founders. They wrote, "Open the back of an expensive watch. Then calmly pour sand right into its delicate works. You wouldn't? Yet your body is the most delicate and valuable machine in the entire world. Then why do millions of people willingly clog it, gum it up?

You're far too intelligent to treat your
body that way ever again."

Switching to Cigars or a Pipe

Other young smokers switch to the pipe. You can
get cancer of the lip and tongue by smoking pipes
for extended periods. But pipes are safer for your
lungs because you do not inhale the smoke. However, it happens to be seven times more dangerous
to use pipes than not to smoke at all. According to
the American Cancer Society, the risk of developing cancer of the oral cavity and esophagus is much
higher for pipe and cigar smokers than for those
who do not smoke at all and approximately at the
same level as for cigarette smokers. The chance of
getting cancer of the larynx is three to seven times
higher for these smokers. Pipe smoking, alone or
with other forms of tobacco use, is also related to
cancer of the lip.

Heavy and prolonged pipe smoking presents
some other dangers. Certain pipes, used over a
long period, often create crooked teeth, for instance. If you keep gnawing the pipe stem—and
you probably will—you can wear down your tooth
enamel. In time, your teeth wind up with some
nasty stains. No toothpaste can remove them.
Chemical irritation and the great heat of lighted
tobacco can also break down the tissues of your

mouth or affect your salivary glands. Likewise, chewing tobacco can do some damage to your body.

There really is no point in substituting any of these for the cigarettes you just gave up.

Marijuana

An estimated fifty million Americans have tried marijuana. One in eleven high school seniors smoke it regularly. More than 50 percent of the juniors have used it. In a Connecticut bust near a public playground, police arrested six kids under ten years old who had smoked marijuana that day. Their elders told authorities not to make such a fuss. The parents themselves enjoyed marijuana along with their friends.

All of this can make you wonder why anyone should worry about marijuana. Most young people have tried it, and after not getting high, never smoked again. Others smoke "grass" only rarely and never achieve that stoned state.

Only a few young adults become potheads. Those few will pay the price of frequent truancy, low grades, and a possible loss of contact with the real world. Some of these constantly stoned people can slide into depression and suffer all kind of anxieties that require the help of a psychiatrist.

Fortunately, pot smoking doesn't become a habit as easily as cigarette smoking. For one thing, marijuana is not physically addictive. (On the plus side, too, you generally suffer few withdrawal symptoms from pot if you quit.)

On the other hand, marijuana is much more expensive than tobacco and less easily available. You can't just wander into your hometown supermarket for a dollar's worth of grass. You need a source who will sell it at ten to thirty dollars a whack. You pay as much (or more) for one marijuana joint as for a whole pack of cigarettes. It is true that you can locate a marijuana seller, but not every young person makes the effort to find one, and the stuff isn't available in every school yard in North America. Because of all this, only the smallest number of people get into the pot scene more than casually. Smoking is just a temporary thing to them, and so they will never develop what doctors call habituation.

There are a few teenagers, however, who work up to seven or more joints a day and then move on to a dependency. These chronic marijuana freaks steer toward a time when they run some serious health risks. According to several reliable medical studies, longtime potheads irritate their valuable lung tissues, so much so that they can suffer the same fate as longtime cigarette smokers. (The spraying of marijuana leaves with chemicals like paraquat makes it more dangerous, of course.) Asthma or chronic bronchitis can be the payoff from smoking too much pot for too long.

The National Institute on Drug Abuse in Washington, D.C., also reports other effects. Marijuana accelerates your heart rate, which can be dangerous for a teenager with inherited heart problems. Smoking over a period of many years can weaken your body's defense system against disease, change your chromosomes, decrease male hormones, and even cause sexual impotence. Chronic grass smokers can end up with cell damage and even brain damage; they may remain "spaced out" for life.

Please note that these perils await only a few persons. However, even if you get really stoned only once and drive a car, you run the risk of getting hurt in an accident and perhaps maiming or

Smoking is for the birds.

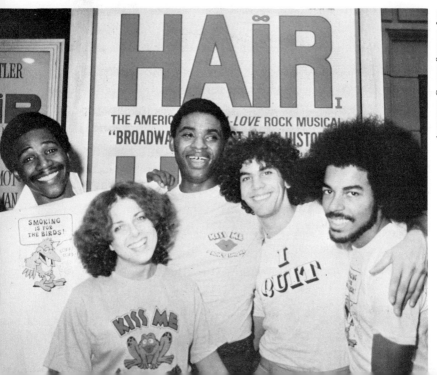

killing someone else. The U. S. Bureau of Narcotics also states that marijuana can lead to heroin use.

Quitting Forever: Becoming an Assertive Nonsmoker

The scene is the elegant Gardiner Tennis Ranch in Scottsdale, Arizona. About eighty people—most of them well-known in the medical, legal, and entertainment fields—assemble to watch the pro's tennis demonstration. It will be followed by a week-long clinic for the paying guests.

One of the guests is a sturdy Kansas boy in his late teens. He has come with his father, a trial judge. Both of the Kansans are nonsmokers.

On a bench directly in front of the two sits a woman of about thirty who has made a name for herself as a movie star. As the tennis pro begins to speak, the actress, out of long habit, lights a cigarette. The smoke drifts directly into the nose of the young Kansan. He hopes that someone will object; after all, the ranch sells a healthful living style. But no one says anything.

After about a minute, the boy takes the initiative. He gently taps the famous film star on the shoulder. "Would you mind," he whispers, "putting out your cigarette? The smoke goes directly into my nose and eyes."

The lady looks up with astonishment, but then

she complies. She is not even offended because it has happened to her before. Nowadays, nonsmokers assert themselves. Most of them, like the boy, do it politely. But they do it.

It has become fashionable to speak up when a smoker annoys you. Teenagers need not hesitate when it comes to tackling their own parents. Some kids have made up signs or billboards with stop smoking messages for the benefit of a mother or father. Other youngsters quietly suggest to a parent not to puff away in the young person's presence.

As we mentioned before, the son of Joseph Califano made his point a few days before his own birthday. When his dad asked about the best birthday gift, the boy said, "This year, I want to ask for something really special."

"Okay, what is it?" the older man said.

"Stop smoking, dad. Do it for me."

It was not an easy task, but Califano followed through. Like most parents, he felt somewhat guilty about smoking. He knew he was setting a bad example for his son. To be sure, teenagers have more clout than they suspect; their elders basically want to be good models for the new generation. If adults continue to smoke, they may indeed lose a young person's love and respect.

Assertiveness makes sense for other reasons as well.

If you happen to be in a closed room with one or

more polluters, you are actually forced to inhale the fumes. This isn't exactly beneficial to your health. According to Hal Higdon, a well-known marathon runner and writer who has done some medical research, a teenager may never become a top athlete if the parents smoked. Here is how Higdon tells it:

> If your father, or particularly your mother, smoked indoors near you during your first six months of life, this probably stigmatized you for life and limited your potential as an athlete in endurance events.
>
> The lungs of newborn children are particularly pliable during this six-month period and will rapidly absorb nicotine from the air. If you happened to be born during the winter, you probably suffered more damage to your pulmonary system because of being forced to remain in the house more. A future long-distance runner with smoking parents loses six minutes from his potential marathon time for each month (of his first six months of life) spent mostly indoors.

Some nonsmokers (or militant ex-smokers) are not afraid of protesting if someone starts polluting the air in an enclosed space. You can protest for important health reasons.

Recent research has shown that someone else's cigarette smoke can make you sick. Remember that sidestream smoke—the smoke from the burning end—has higher concentrations of noxious compounds than the mainstream smoke inhaled by the smoker. The innocent nonsmoker breathes twice as much tar and nicotine in the sidestream smoke as the polluter does. A Harvard medical team found some other truths. If you happen to sit with someone who smokes just seven cigarettes in an hour, you will breathe almost twice as much deadly carbon monoxide than is permitted by industrial plants. The smoke-filled air contains visible smoke particles and invisible gases that may irritate the eyes and nasal passages. These same substances may also trigger allergic reactions.

So it is not surprising that the national Interagency Council on Smoking and Health has stated: "Nonsmokers have the right to breathe clean air, free from harmful and irritating tobacco smoke. This right supersedes the right to smoke when the two conflict."

The trend has swung against the smokers. All kinds of antismoking bills are being introduced in the legislatures of many states. In various polls of the past years, ever more young people made these statements:

- There should be a complete ban of cigarette advertising.
- The U.S. government should not subsidize tobacco farming.
- Cigarette packages should come with even stiffer health hazard warnings.

- Nonsmokers have greater rights than smokers.

Young people have the best chance to change the future of the tobacco industry.

And they no doubt will.

Reading List

Books

Brean, Herbert. *How to Stop Smoking.* New York: Pocket Books, 1970.

Rathus, Spencer A., and Nevid, Jeffrey S. *BT: Behavior Therapy Strategies for Solving Problems in Living.* New York: Doubleday, 1977.

Rogers, Jacquelyn. *You Can Stop.* New York: Simon & Schuster, 1977.

Ross, Walter S. *You Can Quit Smoking in Fourteen Days.* New York: Berkley Publications, 1976.

Shedd, C. W. *You Are Somebody Special.* New York: McGraw-Hill, 1979.

Sobal, Robert. *They Satisfy: The Cigarette in American Life.* New York: Doubleday, 1979.

Booklets, Reports, Magazines

"Your Five-Day Plan" (Booklet, Seventh-Day Adventists, 6840 Eastern Avenue, N.W., Washington, D.C. 20012)

"Teenage Self-Test" (U.S. Department of Health, Education and Welfare, Office on Smoking and Health, Rockville, Maryland 20857)

"Marihuana and Health" (Sixth Annual Report to the U.S. Congress, HEW)

Listen Magazine (6830 Laurel Street, N.W., Washington, D.C. 20012)

"The Smoker's Aid to Non-smoking" (HEW pamphlet, Office on Smoking and Health, Rockville, Maryland 20857)

"The Surprising News about Women and Smoking" (HEW pamphlet, U.S. Government Printing Office, Washington, D.C. 20402)

"The Schick Story" (Pamphlet, Schick Centers, 2917 Fulton Avenue, Sacramento, California 95821)

"Me, Quit Smoking?" (Pamphlet, American Lung Association, Box 596, New York, N.Y. 10001)

"Mind If I Smoke?" (Pamphlet, Pacific Press, Mountain View, California 94040)

Index

155

About the Author

Denver-based Curtis Casewit, a member of the American Society of Journalists & Authors, has written a number of articles about psychology. He helped edit a book about the psychiatric problems of American teenagers overseas. The author of more than twenty books that include the Messner title, *The Complete Book of Mountain Sports*, Casewit is also a translator and teacher.